For Louis

Hugh Fearlessly Eats It All

Cheers!

x

Hugh Fearlessly Eats It All

DISPATCHES FROM THE GASTRONOMIC FRONT LINE

HUGH FEARNLEY-WHITTINGSTALL

BLOOMSBURY

First published in Great Britain 2006
This paperback edition published 2007

Copyright © 2006 by Hugh Fearnley-Whittingstall

The moral right of the author has been asserted

Bloomsbury Publishing Plc,
36 Soho Square,
London W1D 3QY

A CIP catalogue record for this book
is available from the British Library

ISBN 9780747589259

10 9 8 7 6 5 4 3 2 1

Typeset by Hewer Text UK Ltd, Edinburgh
Printed by Clays Ltd, St Ives plc

All papers used by Bloomsbury Publishing are natural,
recyclable products made from wood grown in well-managed
forests. The manufacturing processes conform to the
environmental regulations of the country of origin

www.bloomsbury.com

For Pots and Ivan, who don't mind if they do

ACKNOWLEDGEMENTS

First, a huge thank you to Ruth Metzstein, both for gainful past employment and for invaluable help in choosing and editing this collection. Thanks also to all of the following editors and colleagues past, present and – who knows – maybe future: Lisa Freedman, Aurea Carpenter, Miranda Carter, David Thomas, Shane Watson, Carron Staplehurst, Adrienne Connors, Nicola Jeal, Caroline Roux and Rebecca Seal. At Bloomsbury, thanks especially to Richard Atkinson, Natalie Hunt and Will Webb. And finally, thanks again, as ever, to my agent Antony Topping.

CONTENTS

INTRODUCTION ix

HARD TO SWALLOW 1

I DON'T MIND IF I DO 53

MEAT AND RIGHT 103

TRENDS ON TOAST 151

HOME ON THE RANGE 193

A SLOW HAND 229

HUGH'S QUIZ 273

INDEX 283

CREDITS 287

INTRODUCTION

I am a food writer. Writing about food is what I do – and have done, ever since I left the River Cafe in Hammersmith. That's kind of where, and when, it all began.

I say 'left'. Technically I was fired. It was August 1989, and I had been working there as a sous chef since the beginning of the year. I was having the time of my life, cooking with Rose and Ruth and Sam and Theo, learning all the time about the very best ingredients, about what good meat looks like, and what a box of good tomatoes smells like (intoxicating is the answer – if they don't make you feel ever so slightly queasy, then they are not up to scratch). I was shown how to bone out and 'butterfly' a leg of lamb; how to prepare a squid by pulling out all its milky innards and cutting off the tentacles just in front of its giant, all-seeing eyes; and how to clean a calf's brains, by holding them under a trickling cold tap, peeling off the fine sticky membrane, and running my fingers through the soft crevices to flush out little traces of congealed blood, and the odd tiny shard of fractured skull. This became my favourite job and whenever I had a hangover (which was often) I imagined performing the same cleansing ritual to my own throbbing brain.

Rumours had begun to circulate that someone from the kitchen was going to be 'let go'. Despite being the most popular restaurant in London at the time – as in, hardest at which to get a table – it appeared the business was not prospering. In the restaurant trade the correlation between popularity and profit is not, as I have since had explained to me on numerous occasions, remotely straightforward. It's all about *margins*. These, the accountants had explained to Rose and Ruthie, would have to be increased. Since the restaurant was full every lunch and dinner, since the menu prices were already causing sharp intakes of breath among the diners, not to say lively comment in the press, and since the chef-proprietresses were not prepared to compromise on the quality of the ingredients, the obvious area for cutbacks was staff. The word got out – one from the kitchen and two from front of house were for the chop.

It's hard to explain just how sure I was that the unfortunate sous chef whose release was imminent was not going to be me. It *couldn't* be me. I was just too thoroughly tuned in to what the River Cafe was about. I sniffed the herbs more often, and with louder enthusiasm, than any of the other chefs. I tasted the dishes I was preparing – and those of the other chefs – not once, but several times, arguing (as I still do) that you can't tell if a dish is right until you have eaten a whole portion of it. And when I made a pear and almond tart, or a chocolate oblivion cake, I did so with the undisguised enthusiasm of a greedy child, licking the bowl and the spoon, as my mum had always allowed me to do. At any given time the state of my apron, and my work station, was a testament to my passion. They couldn't possibly fire me. I was having far too good a time!

'The fact is,' Ruthie told me, as we sat on a bench by the Thames that Friday afternoon, 'you're the *least effective member of the team* . . . and . . . *you're slowing everyone else down* . . . and . . . *we're going to have to let you go* . . .'. These harsh words had, I vaguely recall, been prefaced by a kindly, blow-softening preamble extolling the virtues of my enthusiasm and sense of fun, my interest in the ingredients I was cooking with, my good food instincts . . . but none of that really registered. I was too busy being fired – from a job I loved, and hadn't had the least intention of leaving, until it thoroughly suited me to do so. Too busy feeling the injustice – the sheer *wrongness* of the decision. What? No. *No!* Surely I was the *most* effective member of the team, surely I was *geeing everyone else up*, surely they were going to have to let me *stay* . . .

As I began to come to terms with my loss – and it became increasingly clear, from the lack of phone calls begging me to return, that my former bosses were not exactly struggling to come to terms with theirs – I realised I would have to make some big decisions. The looming question to which I rapidly had to find an answer was, 'are you going to get another job in a restaurant kitchen?'

Another way of framing this was, 'Do you really want to be, and have you the talent, determination and discipline to be, a truly great restaurant chef? If not, and given that you've just been fired for being messy and lacking discipline from what is probably the most relaxed and un-hierarchical serious restaurant kitchen in the capital, how much point is there, really, in working in a hellhole dungeon of a kitchen, having your head dunked in the stock pot, being branded with salamanders, and being called a "talentless c**t" a hundred times a day by some cleaver-wielding, caffeine-addicted, ego-maniac chef (mentioning no names) who will happily sacrifice your body, social life and sanity in pursuit of his third Michelin star'. On balance, I thought, not much.

And so I became a food writer.

I am aware that some people are now of the opinion that I have the perfect job. And I am aware that, on all the available evidence, their opinion seems well founded. Writing and broadcasting about something I love, and consequently getting to spend my life discovering it, sampling it, growing it, producing it and consuming it, eventually elicits that embarrassed cliché with which one tries to mask deep smugness with a dose of sarcastic self-effacement: 'It's a tough job, but someone's got to do it. Ha-ha-ha-ha!' Asked recently by another journalist for a one-word description of me, a good friend, after not much pause for thought, I suspect, came up with 'jammy!', and I can hardly disagree.

It's true that I spent the first couple of years of my food journalism career hardly believing my luck. Those very chefs whose tempers and *batteries de cuisine* I knew I could never handle, were inviting me into their kitchens, revealing the secrets of their finest dishes, and feeding me handsomely, all with apparently genuine concern as to my opinion of their craft. And for this, I got paid. Pinch myself? I honestly didn't dare.

Then came the telly. I was introduced to the producer of a Channel 4 show called *Food File*. I told her, half-jokingly, that I felt the show didn't feature nearly enough offal. She told me, half-jokingly, that if I felt so strongly about it, I should present an offal item on the show to make my case. The rest is . . . well, as it happens, bonus material on the *River Cottage Road Trip* DVD.

Ten years later I am still writing and still not infrequently on the telly. I could try and tell you that it is extremely hard work, fraught with identity crises, self-doubts and uncertainties, and loaded with all kinds of pressures and stresses . . . but to expect a sympathetic ear to such pleading – nay, bleating – would be the height of self-absorption, not to say ingratitude. I am, when it comes down to it, so damn jammy you could pile me on a scone and top me with clotted cream.

The mother of an old and dear friend of mine has always referred to pretty much any kind of work in the media, but particularly telly and journalism, as 'showing off'. It's always struck me as a fair cop – both for the profession generally, and for me personally. I think it's helped me to keep a self-critical eye on myself over the years. Because in the end, there is only one conceivable justification for this kind of career choice – for being a 'jammy show off' for a living. It is that those to whom one shows off – one's readers, listeners or viewers – take some net gain from the experience. If you're getting more from it than they are, you're stuffed.

Some perspective is necessary – a desire for world domination is not an essential prerequisite. But there is no shame, I believe, in the ambition to change a small part of the lives of a small number of its inhabitants. And then maybe build on that. Otherwise, frankly, what's the point?

I could hardly claim that changing things and influencing others was my ambition from the beginning. I must admit that when I first declared myself a food writer, I used my job to fulfil a rather selfish wishlist of foodie experiences, from sampling the best food of the best chefs in the UK, to going to Japan to taste sushi right next to the famous Tsukiji fish market.

I hope, and dare to believe, that my work generally, and my writing in particular, has become a little less self-gratifying, and a little more purposeful, over the years. A television audience wants primarily to be entertained – and though one can create a sense of ideology in a show like *River Cottage*, it is books and journalism that give me the opportunity to tell it how I see it on specific issues, and urge others – my readers – to think about things, and maybe, if they start to see the picture differently, do things differently too.

In this collection of my writing, the grounds for inclusion have been along the following lines: a piece made it in if a) it was not so painful and embarrassing for me to re-read that I wanted to run and hide; b) it might conceivably (not necessarily actually) lead to a reader doing something, trying something, saying something, eating something or just thinking something that they might not otherwise have done, tried, said, eaten or thought; and/or c) myself and a coterie of trusted advisers found it passably amusing. You will undoubtedly find articles that would appear to be exceptions to these general criteria, though I guess I could have included anything on the grounds that it might make you think, 'what a waste of space!' or, more specifically, say 'what a tw*t!' out loud.

In the end, if just a few of you find something in this book that resonates or provokes, that makes you angry enough, sad enough, curious enough or excited enough to act on it in some way, then it will all have been worthwhile. The getting fired, I mean.

Hugh Fearnley-Whittingstall
West Dorset, August 2006

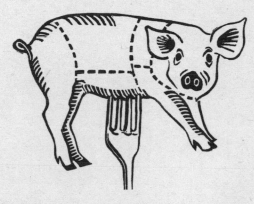

Hard to Swallow

**From corporate crooks to
incompetent cooks …
some food leaves
a funny taste in
the mouth**

This piece was my very first published article (not including student publications). I even got paid for it! I felt like it was a proper journalistic assignment, as it involved 'taking on' one of the great corporate giants, and a certain amount of 'investigative' research, including a visit to a food laboratory.

Okay, it wasn't exactly All the President's Men, but it set, I think, a healthily sceptical tone — about McDonald's in particular, and the fast-food industry in general. It's a theme that I have picked up many times since, and one that — miracles aside — will no doubt demand regular future outings.

Mac attack

Apart from being the longest word in the English language, 'TWOALLBEEFPATTIESSPECIALSAUCELETTUCECHEESE-PICKLESANDONIONSALLINASESAMESEEDBUN' describes perhaps the most remarkable food phenomenon of our time. In common parlance, you know it as the Big Mac.

My assignment: to probe the very essence of its being, and discover its secret. What goes into it? Why do millions buy it? Why do many of the millions actually eat it?

The final challenge: to re-create in an ordinary kitchen, using no industrial machinery of any kind, the precise taste, texture, and unique appearance, of the McDonald's Big Mac.

There are a number of ways of looking at a Big Mac. (With an oblique sideways glance from a distance of at least ten feet has always been my personal favourite.) But, never being one to resist the easy option, I decided to ring McDonald's and ask them straight, 'How do you make a Big Mac?'

'Why do you want to know?' replied the head of PR for McDonald's UK, displaying her verbal fencing skills.

'Well, I'm a freelance food journalist and I want to do a piece on how to make a Big Mac in your own kitchen.'

'Where's the interest in that?'

'I think it would be interesting to see if it could be done.'

'So, what exactly do you want to know?'

'Well, anything. Quantities of ingredients, preparation procedures, cooking times. Everything really. To start with, what are the exact dimensions and weight of the uncooked patties in a Big Mac?'

'I can't tell you that . . . we won't give that sort of information . . . we don't get involved in this sort of thing . . .' and, with a final flourish, 'What I am saying here is that I'm afraid your request falls into the category of being of the kind that we are unable to assist.' Apparently, what she was saying there was that she was afraid that my request fell into the category of being of the kind that they were unable to assist. She had, however, in the course of our conversation, alluded to certain factsheets, available in all the branches of McDonald's, which might tell me more of the things I wanted to know.

In the Chiswick High Road branch of McDonald's I found no such sources of information. 'You mean McFact Cards? We ran out of them weeks ago.' My disappointment was partially offset when I was given an invitation to McHappy Day – until I noticed the date on the invitation: McHappy Day had been and gone, three days earlier.

I finally tracked down some McFact Cards, but they did not exactly tell me how to make a Big Mac. McFact Card No.1 informed me that 'Nowhere in the world does McDonald's use of beef threaten or remotely involve the Tropical Rainforests.' McFact Card No.2 reassured me that McDonald's packaging is ozone-friendly. Finally McFact Card No.3 insisted that 'ONLY prime cuts of lean forequarter and flank are used for our 100 per cent pure beef hamburgers.' Here, at least, was some information I could use.

However, there was something about the way McDonald's were putting themselves across that was beginning to get me down. It was all in that little word *Mc*. McFact, McHappy, McNugget; what the McBloody Hell did it mean? What is a McFact, anyway? Clearly not the same thing at all as an ordinary fact. With this disturbing thought in mind, I decided a more scientific approach was called for.

The next day, at 0900 hours precisely, I visited a McDonald's drive-in, the exact location of which I am unable to reveal. Suffice it to say that this particular establishment is situated not half-a-mile away from an independent food analysis consultancy, whose identity – for reasons of professional etiquette – must also remain secret.

At the drive-in I pulled up, as instructed by the notices, next to a metal grille, which broke the ice by addressing me thus: 'Good morning, we would like to welcome you to McDonald's drive-in.' 'Go on, then,' I thought. But the voice simply asked me for my order. 'Three Big Macs, please.'

'Thank you. Please drive to the first window. Enjoy your meal, and have a nice day,'

I paid at the first window, drove to the second, where a spotty youth explained, 'Your Big Macs are just being prepared, Sir. There'll be a slight delay of a minute-and-a-half.' I received my parcel 86 seconds later.

At 0914 I was handing over my purchase to a man in a white coat. 'They don't smell very nice, do they?' he said, as he removed the first Big Mac from its ozone-friendly container. (This struck me as being a rather unscientific observation, but it was pleasing to have an official confirmation of my own amateur opinion.) The first Big Mac was to be analysed for nutritional content; the components of the second were to be individually weighed to give me my exact recipe; the third was for my breakfast.

My friend in the white coat began the analysis by placing an entire Big Mac into a Magimix, and flicking the switch. In a surprisingly short time, the item was transformed into a smooth and even purée. This substance was remarkably similar in colour, but perhaps marginally thicker in consistency, to a McDonald's chocolate milkshake. Hey McPresto – a Big Mac Shake.

Once the state of the Big Mac had been so radically altered, everything became impressively scientific. Small blobs of the purée were carefully weighed, and placed in test tubes. While one such blob was being mixed with sand, I enquired as to its ultimate fate. 'We burn it overnight at a temperature of 550°C. This gives us the ash content.'

'I should think it does,' I said.

Another blob was to be broken down in a 'Kjeldetherm digester'.

A third piece of purée would spend the afternoon inside a hydrolytic thimble, followed by a whole night in a Soxhlit extractor. Oh, the wonders of modern science.

As all these exciting events were taking place, I turned my attention to the third Big Mac. I had rather lost my appetite. Nevertheless, I felt a tasting at this stage was important, for the sake of experimental propriety. I duly took a (not insubstantial) bite. My teeth fell easily through the layers, apparently untroubled by resistance from any meat-like substance. I was grateful for a small piece of gherkin which got stuck in my teeth. It actually tasted of something.

The following day I received the results of the analysis. A note at the beginning informed me that 'The values obtained were, nutritionally, as expected for this type of product, viz. a good selection of meat, cereal and vegetable protein which could provide the essential amino acids required for growth.' Surely all those horrendous processes to which my Big Mac had been subjected would reveal something more controversial than this? I was consoled by the results of the itemised weighing. At least I now know that a Big Mac comprises 79.4g of bun, 63.6g of beefburgers, 13.2g of cheese, 34.1g of relish and shredded lettuce (a note explained the two were inseparable) and 6.2g of gherkin. It was time to go shopping.

The shopping

First stop, the butcher's, in search of beef-related substances for the patty. In the absence of hard evidence to the contrary, I decided to accept McDonald's specification of 'only prime cuts of lean fore-quarter and flank'. The butcher had an interesting alternative nomenclature: 'Forequarter? Well, we call it "chuck".'

'Sounds encouraging. I'm looking for about a 20 per cent fat content overall.'

'You'll get that with your flank – that's to say, ribs. Very fatty.'

The sundry garnishes, so vital to the final product, might have eluded a less resourceful shopper. Your average processed cheese squares in your average high street supermarket are sadly lacking that science-fiction fluorescent orange glow that characterises the

Big Mac curd factor. I finally tracked down a close approximation in a tiny 24-hour grocer's in the Uxbridge Road. My selection was based on colour-match alone, on the grounds that if the artificial colouring was correct, the artificial taste would naturally (or un-naturally) follow.

I had to visit five delicatessens before I found gherkins of adequate dimensions, i.e. not less than 2.5cm in diameter. For the special sauce I purchased two different types of mayonnaise, two of salad cream, an inferior brand of tomato ketchup, and a small carton of UHT long-life milk, which I felt might be an appropriate thinner. I chose a good firm onion, and a crisp, fresh iceberg lettuce, bearing in mind that it was not their initial state, but the processes to which I would later subject them, that would determine their suitability for inclusion in the end product.

The final shopping challenge was the bun. A particularly tough one to imitate, since McDonald's buns have not two tiers but three, and a distribution of sesame seeds so regular, so mathematical, that I can only imagine they employ cheap foreign labour to stick them on one by one, by hand. Or, perhaps, robots. I eventually plumped for Safeway's 'sesame seeded burger buns' whose sesame pattern and density was relatively uniform, and whose size and colour seemed an excellent match.

Back in my kitchen, I began the patty-simulation phase. This meant throwing my meat into the Magimix and flicking the switch. I watched, transfixed, as the rough hunks of meat slowly transformed, via an intermediate stage of white and rose, into a homogeneous paste of pale coral pink. At this point I formed a little of the mixture into a sort of proto-patty, for a taste test. The resulting mini-burger was disappointing in two important ways: too much texture, and too much taste.

I returned my mincemeat to the Magimix and gave it another two minutes. In the resulting patty I felt I had achieved a close approximation to the original in terms of texture but I still had an excess of flavour on my hands. How do they do it? I wondered. Perhaps McDonald's buy their meat from Bovril, after the beefy flavour has been extracted. I could only hope that 24 hours at minus 16°C would help to chill out some of the remaining flavour.

Although the patty dimensions, cooking procedure and precise recipe for a Big Mac are proprietary information, I had managed to discover, by talking in a childlike manner to a junior member of the McDonald's PR staff, that the precooked weight of each patty was precisely 1.6oz. For those of you at home who lack accurate weighing equipment, it is worth noting that this amount of minced beef will fit very neatly into a standard-size matchbox. As you might imagine, a matchbox of mince spread over an area the size of a burger bun comes out pretty thin. Four millimetres thin, to be precise.

The final dimensions of my hand-moulded imitation Big Mac patties can therefore be revealed (with apologies for mixture of imperial and metric measurements):

Diameter: 11cm (allowing for a ten per cent shrinkage factor)
Thickness: 4mm
Weight: 1.6oz

The McTaste test

The two-man tasting team that gathered around the famous *Punch* table consisted of David Thomas, Editor of *Punch*, and Sean Macaulay, the magazine's lovelorn restaurant critic. Both men were fast food devotees and felt confident that they could distinguish the real McCoy from the McPhoneys.

The two home-made Macs were placed on a tray on which four genuine articles had also been placed. The imitations were remarkably lifelike, but, even so, were soon spotted by the eagle-eyed testers. The give-away was the distribution of sesame seeds; nothing can quite equal the precision with which the Big Mac's seeds are spread around the bun.

On biting into the burgers, Macaulay came over all pretentious: 'The imitation is like a chord – you can taste all the different notes, but they harmonise well together. The real Big Mac is just one great splurge. You can't de-structure it in terms of taste. You can't say, "Oh, there's the cheesy bit."'

For Thomas, the differences were tactile. 'The fake is too solid. I can feel the flour on the bun. There's too much to bite into. A real

Big Mac is squishy. If you put your thumb on the bottom it sinks into the bun. If you take your thumb away, the bun reseals itself. The fake is too real, if you see what I mean. It's a real bun.'

Tastewise, the fake came out way ahead. It was a genuinely delicious burger. Having said that, however, both testers admitted that there was something about the acrid, pickle-y tang of a Big Mac that was, well, McAddictive. There was one other crucial difference: the fake did not produce an afternoon's worth of McFlatulence.

The following is your very own easy-to-follow-cut-out-and-keep-step-by-step guide to cooking a Big Mac at home:

Components

1) The Bun: take your chosen brand of bun and slice it carefully in half. Take a second bun and slice off the top and the bottom, leaving a crustless segment about 8mm in thickness. This will serve as your middle tier. Lightly toast both sides of this tier, and the insides only of the top and bottom tiers, under a hot grill.

2) The Patties: cook your patties from frozen under a maximum heat grill for two minutes on the first side and a minute on the second. You should be aiming for a uniform dark grey/brown colour, both inside and out.

3) The Onions: these should be chopped as finely as possible, approx 1mm x 2mm, and steamed or boiled for at least 15 minutes. They may be kept warm indefinitely.

4) The Lettuce: chop this into shreds of about 3mm in width and 2cm in length. Don't be alarmed if the shredded lettuce is still crisp and crunchy at the time of burger assembly. The heat and moisture of the other ingredients should rapidly achieve the customary degree of flaccidity.

5) The Special Sauce: mix the mayonnaise, UHT milk and ketchup in a 3:2:1 teaspoonsful ratio.

6) The Pickle: you will need two slices of a large gherkin, approximately 1.5mm thick.

7) The Cheese: unwrap one 10cm x 10cm square of processed cheese, ensuring it is the correct Day-Glo orange.

Assembly

1) On the bottom layer of toasted bun, scatter a sprinkling of lettuce, a level teaspoon of onions, and a dab of sauce.

2) On top of this, place your cheese square, making sure the four corners peek cheekily over the side of the bun.

3) Place one hot patty on to the cheese, and press lightly, thereby gently encouraging the cheese to melt.

4) Arrange the middle tier carefully over the first patty and repeat stage 1.

5) Add the two slices of gherkin to this pile, and then mount the second patty on top.

6) Crown lovingly with the bun-cap.

7) The burger should be wrapped tightly in paper and left to 'settle' in a warm tray for at least an hour. (NB This final stage is crucial for authentic results. The ingredients have to coalesce. Subsidence is the key.)

Winter 1989

Over the next decade, McDonald's corporate muscle was exercised in an increasingly heavy-handed manner. Its dubious corporate ethics came under scrutiny during the famous McLibel trial.

It's a McTaste crime

So McLibel is over. No big surprise that three years of legal nit-picking and ten million quid's worth of top silk was enough to raise some reasonable doubt as to McDonald's culpability for most of the various environmental, animal welfare, and nutritional crimes levelled at them by the plucky pair from London Greenpeace. But to those of us who have long been conscientious objectors to McDonald's ruthless global domination of the fast-food market, their recent 'victory' in the courts seems somewhat hollow, not to say Pyrrhic.

The spectacle of the McDonald's legal sledgehammer cracking down on their rather nutty, but undoubtedly principled, accusers, has been pretty unpalatable. So much time and money to refute the allegation that McDonald's is a heartless, greedy, cynical corporate monster, which puts power and profit before environmental responsibility, animal welfare and the nutritional interests of its customers. And so telling that they felt the allegation so badly needed to be refuted.

The libel action, of course, was only part of their defence. It went hand-in-hand with several massive advertising and marketing campaigns, meticulously planned to whip into line wavering loyalty to the product. There was the soppy campaign – shamelessly implying that a trip to McDonald's is a fair substitute for more traditional family expeditions, such as a trip to the zoo or a walk in the park. There was the Space Jam campaign, heralding perhaps the most cynical merchandising alliance of all time, where Bugs Bunny, Michael Jordan, and McDonald's hamburgers were all rolled into one intoxicating package, guaranteed to make a huge impact on impressionable young children, and therefore their parents' wallets. And there is the (most recent) campaign emphasising McDonald's competitive pricing policy with the dubious claim that buying their burgers will actually 'save you money' – not as much money as not buying their burgers will save you, I can tell you.

At the same time McDonald's have launched a kind of in-store Glasnost, so that now you can't get to the service counter without being bombarded by leaflets giving you 'information' about how wonderful they are. The latest of these, a flashily designed colour leaflet dramatically entitled 'Our food: the inside story', contains detailed nutritional information and ingredients lists for every single item on the McDonald's menu. Anybody who can be bothered to plough their way to the end of it might be shocked to discover that McDonald's uses no fewer than 52 E-number additives in their products. Yet the symbolic picture on the front of the leaflet – giving a reassuring subliminal message of unadulterated freshness and health to the many customers who will pick it up, but never read it – is of half a juicy, red, just-cut tomato. And how many of McDonald's products actually contain even the tiniest sliver of a fresh tomato? Not even one!

Still, McDonald's will say, we have nothing to hide – as if by coming clean about all the rubbish they put in their food, they somehow make it more healthy. Putting the upbeat packaging aside, the only reasonable message one could draw from this mass of 'nutritional' information is that McDonald's burgers are probably no worse for you than all the other crap they think you probably eat.

McDonald's has clearly been aware of, and frightened by, the fact that McLibel was alienating a large sector of their potential market in this country. For many of us, their saturation advertising and universal presence on the high street has merely compounded that alienation. In the circumstances, it seems their best defence against serious commercial setbacks has been the zombification of their core clientele. Knowing that a pretty large section of the population is undiscerning enough in its taste, and sufficiently unswayed by issues of food politics to regularly buy their product, their simple mission is now to persuade them, virtually force them, to buy more and more of it. So they hammer home the message, time and time again: McDonald's loves you, and your kids, and you love McDonald's, and so do the kids, and it's dirt cheap, so why don't you just stop thinking about other forms of food and make a pact for eternity that you'll never eat anywhere else?

Just to make it easy for their followers – and this is what I consider to be the *most* offensive of all their publicity offensives – McDonald's will now show them the way to the nearest store, from just about any public place they happen to find themselves. Just follow the arrows on the red and yellow signs, now to be seen whenever one strays within 500 metres of a McDonald's store in the capital – which, let's face it, is just about everywhere one strays. (It is to London Underground's eternal discredit that they have allowed McDonald's to plaster such signs on every single riser of every single step of the exits from numerous tube stations.)

The net result of all this relentless marketing muscle is that either you fall under the McDonald's spell, and herd like sheep into their nearest 'restaurant', or you are forced to conclude that McDonald's really is guilty of some pretty heinous crimes: the calculated narrowing of the nation's culinary options; the deliberate stifling of youthful inquisitiveness about food; and, worst of all, the passing off of something bland, homogeneous and mediocre as something fresh, exciting and essential.

And if they can sell us a lie this big, is there any lie they can't sell us?

July 1997

Seventeen years after first tilting at McDonald's, I was asked to consider whether the massive corporate edifice was finally starting to reveal some cracks.

I'm lovin' it

We all have our fantasy headlines – the announcement of events of global or national significance that chime irresistibly with our own personal values and ambitions. 'Texas oil reserves found to be unlimited' would probably be George Bush's. Though I suppose it might be trumped by 'WMDs found in Iraq – and Iran'.

Well, I almost got to see one of mine this week. 'McDonald's goes bust!' – that would have been the undiluted, full-fat, maximum-caffeine version. In truth the news isn't quite that spectacular. But it's pretty brilliant all the same: 'McDonald's to close 25 stores in the UK'. Yes! For me, and no doubt others who share my loathing of this huge ugly lump of global corporate muscle, this is an air-punching moment. All morning after I heard, I was wandering about in daze of delighted disbelief. And when I'd done with the air-punching, I went for the double forearm salute, shouting 'YES!' again, through clenched teeth, to my two clenched fists. A childish reaction, perhaps, but *schadenfreude* is primordial stuff. And the bigger the beast that's fallen, the greater the glee. In short, I'm lovin' it!

At last, it seems that McDonald's is losing its hitherto stellar domination of the vast fast-food market in this country. This is not a regional or temporary blip, or a mere tactical realignment. They really are in trouble. Their poor performance in Britain dragged profit margins from McDonald's European company-owned restaurants down to 14.9 per cent of sales last year – from 15.6 per cent in 2004. No new openings are planned for the coming year. Even McDonald's European boss, Denis Hennequin, is struggling to put a happy face on the situation: 'The UK has been in negative territory for a couple of years now,' he admitted. 'The brand 15 years ago was very trendy and modern. It is now tired.'

This is dramatic stuff. It was only a few years ago that the march of the Golden Arches seemed inexorable. As recently as 2002 we heard that four new stores were opening somewhere on the planet every day. McDonald's were able to buy the endorsement of any global superstar they felt might enhance their brand. Their supremely aggressive advertising, coupled with relentless merchandising tie-ins with Hollywood blockbuster kids' movies, gave them untold power over the minds, and consequently stomachs, of our kids. They had seemed, for a couple of decades, literally unstoppable. The halting of such a seemingly irresistible force is no mean feat. It smacks of revolution. And as we celebrate (dancing in the high street may not be excessive) we should ask: how has this been brought about?

There's no doubt in my mind that the guests of honour at the big McClosure bash should be Morgan Spurlock, maker of the documentary *Super Size Me*, and Helen Steel and Dave Morris of the McLibel trial, now reworked into a stunning feature documentary. (Incidentally, I think Jamie Oliver deserves a few popped corks, too. McDonald's were not the focus of his school dinners campaign. But they must have suffered by implication.) In the end it is easier for concerned parents to steer their children clear of the Golden Arches than it is for schools to reinvent the greasy wheel of the school canteen. Of course, we all want this to happen, and parental pressure is the only way it will. But it makes sense for parents to put at least some of their money where their mouths are. (In other words, for Turkey Twizzlers read Chicken McNuggets throughout.)

As McDonald's themselves have known for a long time, entertainment is one of the most powerful marketing tools there is – hence Ronald McDonald, and every merchandising deal they have ever done. So to see entertainment used as a weapon against them has been especially satisfying. The two McMovies between them have certainly done a magnificent job of exposing McDonald's as a horrendous corporate bully, and a peddler of nutritionally bankrupt junk.

But much more importantly than that, for my money, is the way they have encouraged us no longer either to fear McDonald's or to genuflect to their supremacy, but to laugh at them. The best piece of pure farce to emerge from the McLibel trial was the revelation that McDonald's had hired at least four private detectives to infiltrate the London Greenpeace campaign group. What's more, not all the investigators were made aware of each other's existence. They therefore ended up wasting fantastic amounts of their time and McDonald's money investigating each other.

Super Size Me, as well as being a sizzling indictment of the devastating effect of the McDonald's diet on the human body, is also a very funny film. And some of its humour is of the gross-out variety so beloved of a teenage audience – Spurlock vomiting up his supersized Happy Meal before he even gets out of the drive-in is practically a Farrelly brothers moment.

Almost as funny as the sight of McDonald's floundering public image is the sight of them trying to do something about it. In their desperate effort to reinvent themselves as a 'healthy option' McD's are doing a grand job of making themselves look ridiculous.

They may for decades have been frighteningly brilliant at selling burgers and fries, but they have, for the past year or so, revealed themselves to be comically bad at selling salads and fruit. According to reports in America, some of their salad meals, once topped with the gunk they call a dressing, contain as much fat as a quarter-pounder with cheese plus a regular fries. If so, that is nothing short of appalling, but it is on balance still funnier than it is sad.

Everyone knows that the best way to disempower the playground bully is to make him a laughing stock. And this, joyfully, is what's starting to happen to McDonald's. This is apt, as it is in the playground that they are most vulnerable. Kids may be easy to reach and influence; showering them with gifts and attention, and glamorous associations with what is cool and happening in their world can be brutally effective. But kids can be ruthless, too, when the lustre of desirability starts to fade, in dropping the stars, the trends

– the brands – they once loved. The most devastating news for McDonald's, and the thing they can do least about, is that they are becoming seriously uncool. A survey published last week revealed that Britain's teenagers are turning their backs on the Golden Arches in droves. Just one per cent of 13- to 15-year-olds said McDonald's was their favourite meal, down seven per cent on a year ago.

We have more to relish here than the satisfying sight of Egg McMuffin on face. The point is not that fast-food culture is on the wane – far from it. In fact, the denting of McDonald's comes at a time when the takeaway sector generally continues to grow. But as it expands it is also diversifying. These days, in the clusters of fast-food outlets in our major cities, we are starting to find, dotted among the big names in burgers, chicken and pizza, some genuine alternatives: the big-name coffee shops, of course, but also juice bars, sushi restaurants, fruit and nut stands, bagel bars, pasty parlours, soup and salad takeaways – and even the occasional organic burger joint. Of course, not all these new ventures are paragons of culinary virtue. Many leave a lot to be desired – some in their trading ethics, others for poor nutrition, or simply a lack of good taste. But it's none the less true that, taking the fast-food sector as a whole, the possibility of an encounter with what we might call 'real food' is definitely on the up.

This is particularly encouraging, not because of any significant change in the sense of where we are now, so much as where we might get to in the not-too-distant future. The fast-food restaurant and takeaway sector has always been a magnet to entrepreneurs. There is clearly an increasing perception among such entrepreneurs that the mood and the opportunities in this sector are changing. In the newest, most innovative forays into fast food – places such as Quiet Revolution, Eat, Love Juice, and Benugo's – there is an emphasis not only on healthy alternatives, but transparency, trace-ability and the provenance of ingredients.

It's tempting to ask, then, whether this is some kind of a tipping point in our food culture. Is it the beginning of the end of the domination of the mediocre, the mass produced and the homo-geneous? Is the tide of junk really turning? Are we as a nation, and is our youth in particular, becoming a little less susceptible to the remorseless clout of marketing megabucks?

To answer a resounding yes would be a touch premature. It's hard to argue that the good food revolution has already achieved an unstoppable momentum, when there are still kids all over the country breakfasting on Coca Cola, crisps and chocolate bars (and there are still schools selling them this crap in their own corridors). Figures on child obesity are still heading up, not down. Most school meals are still are a nutritionally depleted, over-processed disgrace.

But we can at least say that some important messages are starting to get through. In the same survey that saw McDonald's popularity plummet among teenagers, only 12 per cent of 800 comprehensive school students said they did not eat healthily and nearly half of the 13- to 15-year-olds said they ate fresh fruit and vegetables every day, an increase of 14 per cent on last year. McDonald's becoming uncool is obviously a boost to any campaign for better, healthier eating. But the idea that fresh fruit and vegetables might actually become cool for kids is, in the long term, even more exciting.

For me, the biggest boost to come from the news about McDonald's is that it gives heart to other campaigns that strive to liberate our food culture from, arguably, even more powerful corporate beasts. Today the real stranglehold comes not from the behemoth fast-food brands, but from the big four supermarkets: Tesco, Morrisons, Asda/Wal-Mart and Sainsbury's. Between them, they control 75 per cent of the grocery market in the UK. There are hundreds of thousands of farmers and food producers, here and all over the world, selling groceries to tens of millions of British shoppers. Yet the growing, processing, distribution and sale of all that food is controlled by just four companies. That has to be unhealthy. If it wasn't for the tremendous diversity, commitment, passion and creativity that is, against all the odds, being preserved in the small fraction of the market they do not yet control, you could say that the supermarkets *own* our food culture.

For me, then, the true tipping point will come when significant numbers of consumers begin to say to the supermarkets: Enough of your bullying tactics to farmers and producers, your misleading labelling and spurious nutritional information; Enough of the systematic suffering of livestock in intensive systems, driven by you, as you push the price points lower and lower; Enough of your dirty, polluting, wasteful food miles, and your outrageous, undemocratic flouting of planning law and the opinions of local people.

The way to do this effectively is to change the way you shop. You don't have to stop going to supermarkets, but you do have to take from their shelves only those products you believe are honestly and ethically traded, transparently labelled, environmentally sustainable, and not abusive of either animals or people. And go elsewhere for the rest.

This is a lot to ask of the nation's shoppers, and until recently the possibility of bringing about genuine change in the dominant food retail culture seemed fanciful. Raising a groundswell of popular opinion to question the supermarkets' methods, their ethics and the true value of their contribution to our society felt like a hopeless task. But now, with Britain's unambiguous backlash against McDonald's giving hope to this campaign, nothing seems impossible. Things are already hotting up on the battleground. Will Tesco try to sue the Tescopoly activists and embarrass themselves, McLibel style, in the process? Will the Wal-Mart film, *The High Cost of Low Price*, prove to be the *Super Size Me* of supermarket culture, helping to deflate, and ultimately disarm, another mighty corporate bully?

Let's hope so. Because if such once unimaginable events do occur, I might just get to see one of my other fantasy headlines: 'Tesco in turmoil! Shoppers desert supermarkets for born-again high streets.'

March 2006

And if Ronald McDonald is a cynical creation, then KFC's pseudo-curmudgeonly Colonel really takes the patty . . .

Giving the Colonel his marching orders

At one time I wasn't entirely sure whether or not Colonel Sanders, the face of Kentucky Fried Chicken, was a real person. In fact he was: Colonel Harland Sanders, to give him his full title, was born in

Indiana in 1890, though he didn't begin his business of franchising fast-food outlets for another 65 years. I guess he was a late starter, and I've nothing against that. But to my mind it's a pity his post-pensionable energies weren't spent on some gentler pursuit. Because the Colonel was the principal pioneer of a range of products that rightly came to be known as junk food. And behind the global success of his brand is an enormous and revolting industry: the factory farming of poultry. The fact is, without Colonel Sanders, we might never have had Bernard Matthews. And for that alone he deserves our deepest resentment.

If the litmus test for the ethics of any farming method lies in the behaviour of the animals within the system, then factory farming of poultry is probably the least defensible kind of meat production. It drives the chickens in question to aberrant, utterly unnatural behaviour. To begin with, we're talking about thousands of chickens crammed into a shed. And not just any chickens, but a strain that has been bred genetically to be obese. Left to its own devices scuttling around a farmyard, a chicken would take around four to five months to get to a decent size for eating, but the industry can now get a bird to this size in just under six weeks.

That's if they live that long. Mortality in intensive broiler houses runs at a standard seven to ten per cent (which means around five to seven million birds in the UK are dying prematurely), not least because of the phenomenon known in the industry as a 'smother'. This occurs when the birds get so stressed out – perhaps the temperature control goes a bit haywire, or the ammonia levels from the deep litter (which, incidentally, isn't changed for the whole of the six weeks of their life) gets too high – that they think 'we can't take this anymore' and make a kind of suicidal rush in one direction, piling on top of each other to lethal effect.

This makes nonsense of the marketing of the Sanders character, which is all about just how generous the Colonel is, with his Bargain Buckets and his special crispy coating. In terms of distracting the consumer from the actual story behind the food in the shop, he's up there with Ronald McDonald. It's a classic conjuring trick: let's get everyone to look in this direction – where we are waving and shouting about the idea of a bib-and-tucker, hearty, down-home

American meal – while backstage in the secret compartment there is a highly abusive, morally abhorrent industrial farming process going on. It can only be hoped that last week's disgusting revelations – about conditions inside the West Virginia plant of a former KFC 'Supplier of the Year', where live birds were filmed being spat on, tortured and smashed against walls – will make this trick more difficult to pull in future.

The Colonel's own iconic image has evolved over the years, beginning as a fairly realistic silhouette based on a genuine photograph, but ending up as a cartoon. This summarises the evolution of his product, which itself has become more plastic and malleable as the raw ingredient has got less and less like real chicken. One has to ask the question, wouldn't it actually be simpler to make the fast-food product out of the same stuff as the chicken feed? There's little doubt that soya technology could now simulate the flavour and texture of Kentucky Fried Chicken without actually troubling a real bird to produce the substance of the dish.

It might ease the sense of outrage to hear that Colonel Sanders wasn't entirely happy about what was done in his name, but he remained the public face of the company until his death in 1980. So the individual as well as the icon has to take a share of the blame. It was the man himself who put into place the systems that shift such high volumes of chicken, stimulating the entrepreneurs of industrial farming to concentrate on ever cheaper and more efficient ways of producing chicken flesh.

Now the icon has long since transcended the man, and it is this grinning, paternalistic, pseudo-curmudgeonly cartoon face that fills me with such rage. Somewhere between Father Christmas and Abe Lincoln, it seems designed to assuage any public anxiety about the origins of the product before any serious questions can be asked. To me it has a vile aura. The more I see it, the more I want to smash it with my fist.

July 2004

In terms of blighting our food culture with its perniciously pervasive tendrils –
and therefore generally getting my goat – the only thing that gives the fast-food
industry a run for its money is the diet-food industry. Here goes . . .

Dr Death rides out

I know one is not supposed to speak ill of the dead, but Dr Atkins –
what a wanker! I say this only partly because I am sick of wading
through a list of 17 books apparently written by him (the Atkins
brand gives new meaning to the phrase 'ghost writer') before I even
get close to any book of my own in the Amazon Food and Drink top
100. I say it only partly because I realise that his influence over the
eating habits of the nation exceeds mine by a factor of squillions. And
I say it only partly because I am affronted by the sheer jaw-dropping
gall of churning out books like bank notes, all of which say precisely
the same thing, something that could anyway be summarised in ten
words: 'Ditch the starch. Stuff your face with meat and fat.'

I insist that jealousy is but a piquancy in the rich, heady mixture of
negative emotions, the Angostura bitters in the overall cocktail of
rage, that I feel whenever the name of Atkins and his bloody diet
comes up. What really gets my goat is something far more irritating
than its colossal success, or even the fact that it actually seems to
work. What bugs the hell out of me is the widespread myth that the
Atkins diet is somehow gastronomically generous or enlightened;
that it allows those who follow it to eat good food – in either the
sensual or the physically virtuous sense of the word.

Someone put this notion to me pretty bluntly the other day.
'You'd love the Atkins diet,' they said. 'Why?' I said, brow
furrowing, fists involuntarily clenching. 'Because he says everyone
should eat loads of meat and fat and butter and cheese. And that's
what you like eating the most, isn't it?' The answer is that I do like
these things. But I like them in context. I like them in conjunction
with, though not necessarily at the same time as, a lot of other foods
– in particular fresh fruit and vegetables.

Consider the ruthless cynicism of what Atkins has achieved. It has
long been the diet peddler's best ruse to concoct a programme that

can claim it is not based on denial – that insists you can rapidly lose weight and still eat the things you really like. This myth is what those absurd and revolting products such as fat-free cakes and artificially sweetened fizzy drinks are all about. If you can shut down your taste buds, cancel your gag reflex, and think of the adverts and packaging, you might just be able to imagine you're having a treat.

Atkins has gone one further, or even two or three further. It's not just that he allows you the occasional indulgence. He takes the one substance that dieters fear most, and miss most – FAT – and effectively encourages them to eat it to the exclusion of most other foods. He might as well have called the diet Binge Yourself Thin.

It has been pointed out by many critics of Atkins that one should not confuse a successful weight loss programme with healthy eating, and that however effective the diet is in busting blubber, it is certainly not good for you. In fact, it is almost self-evidently true that any rapid weight loss programme can hardly be healthy. You can of course lose weight by starving yourself completely – and shed a couple of extra ounces by cutting off your nose to spite your face.

Well, neither should one confuse a generous allowance of meat and saturated fats with unrestrictive gourmet dining. In fact there is plenty of privation in the Atkins diet. Plenty of good food, again in both senses, is banned. Fruit, for example, is banned for the first few weeks of the diet, and strictly limited thereafter. This has rightly appalled nutritionists, who understand that fresh fruit is perhaps the most accessible key to healthy eating – a potential life-saver for millions.

The fruit ban appals me, however, not as a nutritionist, but as a sensualist. The flavours and aromas of fresh fruit are among the highest pleasures of the table. Think of our English strawberries, for which we just had such a fine summer, and the fresh zesty flavour of our apples, pears and plums, which are just coming on line now. Yes, it's great to have some cream with your strawberries, and perhaps a slice of Cheddar with your apple. But give me a choice between the fruit and the fat, and I'd take the fruit any day.

And what of the meat, for which the Atkins dieter is encouraged to develop such a voracious appetite? As it happens I am currently writing a book about meat. Could be zeitgeisty, you might think. A useful handbook for the millions of Atkinsites currently indulging the pleasures of the flesh.

But I am revolted by the Atkins take on meat. My argument is that we should respect meat, and the animals from which it comes, and do it, and them, justice by choosing it wisely, and using it well. I suggest that, as an ideal, we should all be ready to pay more money to eat less meat, of better quality, from happier animals.

Meanwhile Atkins is turning meat into a food lacking all dignity – a pappy filler for cheated appetites and a junk medicine for human vanity. Eat a cow and lose a kilo. It puts meat on a par with Diet Coke, and it doesn't get any worse than that.

The one known side-effect of the Atkins diet is that it makes your breath smell like hyena poo, which at least makes it easier to identify and remonstrate with offenders. The jury's still out on whether it will give you cancer and/or heart disease. But if, as nutritionists fear, the intrinsic lack of balance in the diet increases the likelihood of these and maybe other fatal diseases, then I guess the small matter of becoming a gastronomic philistine into the bargain may seem insignificant. But it matters to me.

Hugh's anti-Atkins diet

This is principally a diet for energy and health, not weight loss, but serious fatties will probably find the kilos fall off. By rights I should earn billions for this, as it is guaranteed to keep you well-nourished and fit for the rest of your life. But here it is, gratis, from the goodness of my happy, healthy heart:

For breakfast

Eat a bunch of fresh fruit. Then, if you're still really hungry, have a piece of toast.

Mid-morning snack

Eat more fruit. Then, if you're still really hungry, have another piece of toast.

Lunch

Eat a bunch of veg. Raw if possible. If you're still hungry, have a sandwich (but not two), or a piece of chicken, or a lump of cheese (but not both). Eat with juice or water, not Coca Cola or Fanta.

Mid-afternoon

Have another piece of fruit. If it's a bad day, have a biscuit too.

Supper

Eat whatever the hell you like. If you're actually trying to lose weight, eat whatever the hell you like, but not too much of it.

September 2003

Fat-free . . . and slightly lacking in the brain department too . . .

What is the most meaningless phrase in food marketing? My personal vote would be, '92 per cent fat-free' (or any other per cent, come to that). Anyone who thinks this statistic says anything either useful or good about a food product is at best gullible, at worst an idiot (and, quite likely, a gullible idiot).

Of course the implication of the 'fat-free' slogan is that the food so labelled can be eaten in large quantities without any adverse effect on your weight or your waistline. This has to be the biggest, nay fattest, lie the bow-tie-and-big-glasses brigade have ever come up with – not a bad accolade for a profession whose sole business it is to tell porkies to the public.

To emphasise just how absurd it is, here is a list of foods that are 100 per cent fat-free. Just ask yourself how sensible it would be to eat a kilo of any of these for breakfast:

Raspberry jam

Golden syrup

Chilli powder

Salt and vinegar (without the chips)

Sherbet lemons

Vitamin C

Neurofen

Bonemeal

Charcoal

. . . I could go on.

It is, of course, partly a problem of language. The word that describes a whole family of oily hydrocarbons that feature prominently in the composition of all living matter, both plant and animal, and are absolutely essential for human health, just happens to be the same word we use to describe people who are somewhat larger than they (or we) would like to be. Because few of us actually want to be 'fat' (the pejorative adjective), and because the consumption of large amounts of 'fat' (the neutral noun) has been identified as just one possible cause of people becoming 'fat' (the PA), 'fat' (the NN) has been completely demonised.

Meanwhile the demonisation of fat has become a wonderful smokescreen that allows the food industry to dump all sorts of other rubbish in their products for slimmers. It is the marketing equivalent of the crudest, oldest conjuring trick there is – provided you make the audience look intently at your right hand you can get up to all sorts of tricks with your left. Take a look at the ingredients list (you'll need a magnifying glass) of any biscuit, cake, chocolate bar or treat product that is emblazoned with some kind of fat-free, reduced-fat or low-fat slogan boast, and just count the amount of refined sugars, invert syrups, humectants, emulsifiers and preservatives they contain.

The trick for the manufacturers of these products is to work out at what percentage point the fat-free figure will fail to impress its target market, as it begins to dawn on them just how idiotic the whole scam is. So where would you draw the line? 87 per cent fat-free? 82 per cent? 77? 51?

To get things in perspective, let's consider Nigella's chocolate brownies, a recipe from *Domestic Goddess* that almost on its own excuses her dire last book and series. They are superbly rich and delicious, as chocolatey, gooey and indulgent as any fantasising slimmer, or out-and-out greedy guts, could ever wish for. Well, I've been busy with the calculator and worked out that this sublime confection is, astonishingly, an impressive 71 per cent fat-free! By the time you've factored in the calories you will burn up beating the eggs into the mixture, walking around the kitchen picking up ingredients and bending over a few times to open and close the oven door, you can rest assured that a couple of Nigella's brownies will be a far healthier contribution to your diet, and infinitely more of a treat, than any additive, addled 'treats' the slimming industry can offer you.

Interestingly, McVities have recently dropped the 'fat-free' splash on their range of cakes and biscuits for slimmers – perhaps because they finally realised what an insult it was to the intelligence of their customers. What a shame they didn't have a rethink on their brand name as well. If anything it's even more insulting, and it gets more and more irritating every time you hear it. Go ahead!, my arse. What could be more cynical? They realise of course that what slimmers want more than anything is permission to eat the sugary treat foods that the diet books, slimming clubs and other waistline mentors are constantly telling them to steer clear of. So their brand name is nothing less than an imperative exhortation to those struggling with their conscience to simply give in to it: Go ahead! Stuff your face!

I don't mind betting that most slimmers who have decided to make the Go ahead! products part of their weight-loss programme have actually put on weight. How could they not? Every time they open the cupboard door there is a packet of biscuits winking at them saying 'Go ahead! Go ahead! Go ahead!' If I had my way McVities would be forced to rename the entire range, 'Go ahead – eat the whole fucking packet you greedy pig! And then wonder why you didn't just buy a Mars bar in the first place!'

No doubt the products were launched – some years back now – in supermarkets across the nation, by fit-looking young guys and girls dressed in the green and gold livery of the product, carrying plates of the cakes and biscuits around the store, and accosting any customers who looked like they had a few spare pounds around the middle, with a winning smile and warm entreaty to 'Go ahead!' And no doubt few could resist the offer of a guilt-free treat.

Imagine if they had the nerve to turn up again in the supermarkets now, having encouraged would-be slimmers all over the country to simply pile on the pounds. Faced with same obsequious smile, and the same earnest invitation to 'Go ahead!', what self-respecting fatty could honestly resist the temptation to punch them squarely on the nose? Surely no jury would convict?

Quadruple chocolate chip cookies

This is my personal contribution to the pantheon of recipes to help people lose weight. The finished biscuits are about 73 per cent fat-free. And of course, like all slimming products, the more you eat, the thinner you get.

Makes 20–30 cookies

100g soft unsalted butter; 100g caster sugar; 100g soft brown sugar; 1 egg; 125g self-raising flour; 50g cocoa powder; 100g ground almonds; 50g plain chocolate chips; 50g milk chocolate chips; 50g white chocolate chips

Cream the butter and both sugars until soft and whippy. Beat in the egg and then mix in the flour and cocoa, then the ground almonds. Mix in the chocolate chips.

With floured hands, roll chunks of dough into walnut-sized balls. Place them well-spaced apart (they will spread out a lot) on to greased, floured baking sheets or non-stick parchment. Bake at 180°C/Gas mark 4 for 12–15 minutes, until golden brown.

Eat while still warm and soft, or wait until cooled, and more crispy.

January 2004

While some companies boost their profits by ruthlessly exploiting the consumer's fear of fat, others are in the business of selling fat itself. Naturally they are quick to tell us just how healthy it can be, when it's the right kind of fat. But should we believe them?

Taking sides in the fat wars

Those who take the blindest bit of notice of advertising hoardings may have clocked the fact that next Sunday more people throughout Britain will be jumping up and down in unison than have ever done so anywhere in the world. You may well ask, 'Why?' Perhaps the truest answer is, 'so Van den Bergh Foods Ltd, the makers of Flora, can sell more of its margarine'.

Flora, the best selling margarine in Britain, is the official sponsor of the Aerobathon, in which a total of 140,000 people are expected to jig, bounce and sweat, in six of the country's biggest indoor arenas, to live music played by the likes of D:Ream, E17, Kim Wilde and Gary Glitter.

But the aerobists are not the only ones bouncing and sweating. The people at Van den Bergh have been increasingly jumpy since a series of recent studies have introduced a new ingredient into the debate about fats in our diet.

The latest buzz-phrase, which takes its place alongside high cholesterol and saturated fats in the chamber of dietary horrors, is 'trans-fatty acids'. The fats are produced by the process of hydrogenation, in which liquid oils are superheated to produce hard fats, which are blended with liquid oils to make a spreadable product. Almost all margarines and low-fat spreads contain trans-fatty acids. They also occur naturally, in smaller quantities, in animal fats.

Last year Walter Willet, Professor of Nutrition at Harvard University, published a paper based on a study of the diets of 85,000 American nurses, and demonstrated a direct link between trans-fatty acids in the diet and heart disease. Almost all nutritionists now accept that trans-fatty acids increase the level of 'bad' cholesterol. What is claimed by an increasing number of nutritionists is that the trans-fatty acids produced by hydrogenation are qualitatively different from those that occur naturally, and may be much worse than either animal trans-fats or saturated fats.

Udo Erasmus, a Canadian nutritionist, is St George to the Dragon of trans-fatty acids. In his book, *Fats that Heal and Fats that Kill*, just published in America, he lays a catalogue of health problems at the door of these hard fats, citing studies that link trans-fatty acids with PMT, mastalgia (breast pains), impaired muscle tone, kidney dysfunction, high blood-pressure, numerous allergic reactions, and even decreased testosterone.

Van den Bergh, which also makes Delight, Outline, Blue Band, Stork and Echo, is keen to play down the adverse effects of trans-fatty acids. According to Dr John Brown, director of the Flora project for heart disease prevention: 'There are many inaccuracies being put about over trans-fats, mainly by people with an interest in damaging the image of brand leaders like Flora. It's not true, for example, that the trans-fats that occur naturally in animal fats are less harmful than the ones produced by hydrogenation.'

'Oh, yes, it is,' says Simon Wright, a food technologist. 'The kind of fats we are putting in our body when we eat margarine have only been around for 20 or 30 years, since hydrogenation was invented. I'm not happy about that, because I'm not convinced that the long-term effects of eating these artificial substances manifest themselves that quickly.'

Wright is not selling butter. He is, however, selling a product called Superspread, made by Whole Earth, one of only two spreading-fat products on the market that are entirely free of trans-fatty acids (the other is called Vitaquell).

You don't need Jeremy Paxman to set these two camps in combative mood. Van den Bergh foods says it is not possible to make a spread that is low in saturates without using at least some trans-fatty acids. Whole Earth says it is, and it has done it. Van den Bergh says that Superspread is too oily, and would not be acceptable to its consumers. Whole Earth says that is just a gripe, because its process is patented, and cannot be used by Van den Bergh.

Nor is this just a battle of words. Van den Bergh foods recently complained to the Advertising Standards Authority about a full-page advertisement taken by Whole Earth, which opens with the assertion that 'trans-fats may be the biggest single health hazard of our time'. The ASA has yet to make a ruling in this case.

But in the margarine war, Van den Bergh is taking no chances. Flora has recently been reformulated, and the level of trans-fats reduced from 8g per 100g to 1.5g – one of the lowest figures for any margarine. Consumers of Flora may have noticed a corresponding softening in texture, but they received no explanation for this change, on the pack or in advertising. And why, if trans-fatty acids are no worse for you than saturated fats, was a new recipe called for?

Dr Brown is adamant that trans-fats were not the issue in the reformulation: 'The aim was simply to bring down the overall proportion of saturated fats plus trans-fats – this is the nutritionally important figure. It just happened that, for technical reasons, in trying to get the right quality, the trans-fats came down, and the saturated fats went up by a little bit.' Odd, though, that in on-pack labelling terms, Flora now appears to be less healthy than before, since the well-known baddies, saturates, have gone up – from 13.5g per 100g to 17g.

On the other hand it must be a comfort to Van den Bergh to know that, should further research confirm nutritionists' worst fears about trans-fats, Flora's bow-tie boys will be able to say, with some self-satisfaction, 'Well, of course we reduced the level of trans-fats in Flora by over 80 per cent back in 1994.'

Dr Brown insists: 'That's not why we did it.'

It is understandable that Van den Bergh should be reluctant to claim credit for 'taking action' over trans-fats. It would be admitting it has a problem. Rather than publicly entering a gloomy scientific debate, their strategy has been to strengthen the brand leadership of Flora with aggressive, and expensive, marketing. Hard on the heels of the Aerobathon comes an up-beat new advertising campaign. A series of billboard posters, featuring tanned bodies daubed in body paint with the Flora sunflower logo, will seek to refix the glue on the public's association between Flora margarine, and health, fitness and the body beautiful.

There is no denying the power of the campaign. The 'image' magazine *Creative Review* describes it as 'a sexy signal to consumers and a war-like defence of brand leadership'. In one image the body paint spells 'working man', and depicts a window on the model's chest through which are seen cogs and wheels, suggesting a role for Flora as some lubricating panacea of the human system. Another slogan is simply, 'Sunflower Power'. Splashed across the torso of an airborne youth, long golden locks flying, it brings the rave generation into the Flora fold.

This will be a major body-blow to Flora's competitors. And it serves as a strong reminder that there are two battlegrounds in the Fat Wars. A lost skirmish in the nutritionist's laboratory may count as nothing, compared to a flamboyant victory in the media of mass advertising.

April 1994

Dog's breakfast

Anyone who has not yet abandoned their New Year's health drive may have found themselves experimenting, in the last few weeks, with the range of supposedly 'healthy' snacks, that have for some time now been nestling alongside the chocolate bars in sweet counters up and down the land.

Most prominent among these at the moment is Kellogg's Nutri-Grain bar, a product which is being marketed not just as a healthy low-fat snack but as a genuine alternative to breakfast. You've probably seen the boxes of bars lined up right next to the till in your local newsagent – the result, no doubt, of heavy pressure exerted by Kellogg's ruthless team of sales reps. And you can't have missed the New Year saturation poster campaign, with its slogan, 'Go fat out all day!' and its claim that Nutri-Grain bars are '92 per cent fat-free'. So perhaps, like me, you've finally succumbed to the pressure, and actually bought and eaten one.

Can you believe how disgusting they are? The one I chose purported to be blueberry flavoured. Just opening the blue foil wrap released a pungently sweet and artificial smell, like a car air freshener vainly trying to cover up the odour of fresh baby sick.

I dared to risk a bite, and found the coating, which looks like a biscuit, turns out to be soft, soggy and insipid, like the outside of a stale fig roll. And the so-called blueberry filling tastes like second-rate jam, of the kind last encountered inside another highly questionable product, the Pop-tart, also made by Kellogg's.

I only managed one mouthful, which I foolishly swallowed, before quickly deciding that the bar should be renamed Putri-Grain. If this is supposed to be a slimming aid, then it can hardly help that it makes you crave a large bacon butty just to take the sickly aftertaste away. Breakfast? I wouldn't feed one of these to my dog – unless I wanted to punish him, or purge him.

As for the '92 per cent fat-free' claim, that is, of course, just another way of saying that these bars are 8 per cent fat. A look at the label reveals that the fat in question is 'hydrogenated vegetable oil', a chemically refined substance now believed by many nutritionists to be at least as harmful as hard animal fats such as butter.

I never expected to like the Nutri-Grain bar. But I certainly didn't believe it would turn out to be this vile. Here is a product that truly deserves to fail and fail miserably, because not only is it utterly disgusting to eat, not particularly good for you (compared, say, to fresh fruit or unadulterated whole grain cereal); it's not even original. An American health food company called Barbara's have been making (genuinely) fat-free, fruit-filled cereal bars for years. They're made with organic whole wheat and no refined sugar (as opposed to the ordinary refined wheat flour and sugar used by Kellogg's in the Nutri-Grain bar), but, more importantly, they're actually quite pleasant to eat. Incidentally, you won't find them by the till in your nearest newsagents or corner shop, but they are available in most health food stores.

One can be sure that Kellogg's, having invested so heavily in the product, plan to make a fight of flogging us this second-rate pap. But if the Nutri-Grain bar is still on the shelf in two years' time, then I for one will feel an important battle has been lost in the war to uphold sound value and good taste in the face of corporate muscle in the food market.

January 1998

Sadly, a whole decade later, Kellogg's Nutri-Grain is still available. A year or two back, they announced a new recipe for the bar. In the interests of research, I tried another one. It was every bit as revolting as the first . . . possibly more so.

The sour taste of sweet FA

On Sunday I had a truly horrible experience. Half a dozen of us were watching football at a friend's house, when one of the girls sat down next to me with a large tumbler, chinking with ice. 'What have you got there?' I asked, feeling a thirst gathering around my gums. '*Ri-bee-na*,' she said, looking at me wide-eyed with mock seduction, 'do you *want* some?' Yes, I wanted some.

I was pretty parched, and the initial wetness and coldness of the drink was pleasant enough. But within seconds things started to go wrong. The anticipated flavour and satisfaction were not forthcoming. The promised sweetness, the flavour of real blackcurrants, the reliable delivery of refreshment to the back of the throat, all eluded me, as my tongue made a vain search around my mouth for the familiar taste, so comforting in childhood, of good old Ribena.

I was left with a nagging, insipid irritation, which half dared me to take another sip. But I knew I didn't want to, because I realised what had happened: this was not real Ribena, this was Ribena Lite.

It's not a new product, but it is one I had steadfastly managed to avoid – until Sunday. Now that I have tasted it, I can only say I feel polluted – it's such an unpleasant drink, it really shouldn't be allowed to go out under the same name as the original. But then I feel the same way about Coca Cola (an undeniably great drink) and Diet Coke (an abomination). The common ingredient, of course, is the artificial sweetener, aspartame. I absolutely loathe the stuff.

Whenever I taste these, or any other, artificially sweetened drinks (almost always by accident) I am at a loss to explain how popular they have become. They are so . . . *nothing*. The 'taste' of these products is a chimera, a chemical illusion of sweetness: just when you think you might catch it on your tongue, it disappears into a flavourless black hole. The drinking experience is empty, unfulfilling, a sensational void. As Tony Curtis said, after kissing the aptly named Sugar Kowalczyk (Marilyn Monroe) in *Some Like It Hot*, it's 'like smoking without inhaling'.

In the movie of course he was pretending, to get more. But off set Curtis was less than complimentary about Marilyn's oral commitment. He is rumoured to have described the snog as 'like kissing Hitler'. Actually I feel the same way when I take a sip of a diet drink – a substance from which all civilised values have been extracted – because the artificial sweetener that replaces nature's sugars has become one of the Great Dictators of modern consumerism.

The drinks companies like to call these products 'sugar-free' or 'lite', but in truth there is nothing 'free' about them, and I find the whole business heavily disturbing. They are selling cans of nothing – fizzy water with a few unpleasant chemicals added. Yet bolstered by some of the flashiest, most expensive propaganda in the Western world, they have somehow become a force, en-slaving millions of anxious calorie-counters in the polymer chains of these artificial substances.

Converts to the sugar-free life (and there are a scary number of them) have a habit of getting all evangelical on me. 'Keep trying it,' they tell me, 'you'll get used to it', or, 'everyone resists at first'. These exhortations to overcome my aversion and 'join the club' are not appreciated. Truth be told, they make my flesh crawl. I start to feel like Donald Sutherland in *Invasion of the Body Snatchers*: the last sane person in a swelling mob of zombies.

But I won't give in. They won't get me . . . they won't I tell you . . . please . . . NO . . . AAAAARRGH!

October 1997

Sweets gone sour

Of course some foods would never pretend to be healthy, and would rapidly lose their following if they did. I went on my own to the cinema last week, and decided to choose for company a few old friends from the 'pick and mix' sweet shop in the Odeon Marble Arch: toffee bonbons, wine gums, and American hard gums.

They were, in every case, extremely disappointing, compared to my youthful recollection of them. Worst, perhaps, was the toffee bonbon. A good one, I seemed to recall, has a real toffee in the middle, so that after a few chews the sugary coating dissolves away and you are left with a decent bit of buttery toffee between your teeth. In the case of the ones I bought at the Odeon there was only coating: once this had cracked and crumbled to sugary dust in your mouth, there was nothing left to chew on but a sickly aftertaste.

The other sweets were not up to scratch either: both the toffee and chocolate in the eclairs were sub-standard, the wine gums lacked acidity, and the hard gums were, well, not hard enough. I was beginning to wonder what the problem was. Did my youthful memory deceive me, or do they just not make them like they did in the old days?

After the film I went back to the shop to check on the progeny of what I had bought. All the sweets were credited to a company called Tudor Confectionery, and I at once realised the problem. This is a case of licensed plagiarism, like the old *Top of the Pops* records, where the hits of the day are recreated not by the original artist but by some hopeless untalented wannabee.

For the record, a quick bit of research in my local sweet shop reassuringly confirmed that Trebor still make the original and best toffee bonbons, Maynards the *only* acceptable wine gums and hard gums, and the finest chocolate eclairs, with real chocolate and toffee. It is no credit to Odeon Cinemas that they accept Tudor's pale imitations.

January 1998

Travel provides the opportunity for all kinds of exciting and memorable food encounters – some of the best of which are described in the next chapter. But, from time to time, it inevitably puts one at the mercy of one's hosts – in the broadest sense – and that can be memorable for all the wrong reasons . . .

Tunnelling new depths

What's the single most exciting British engineering project of the past 50 years? To be honest, that's not the kind of question I would normally grace with an answer, not being an exciting-engineering-project kind of guy. But there is one thing that has made a deep and lasting impression on me, not least because I have a French girlfriend, and consequently it has had an impact on my whole life. I'm talking, of course, about the Eurostar. I love and adore it.

I love the glass dome at Waterloo. I love the incredible efficiency and politeness of the staff in the ticket office. I love the concourse beyond the ticket barriers, with its excellent little bookshop. I love the escalators and walkways, sensibly signed so that you end up with minimal effort at exactly the right part of the train. I love the reversible yellow and blue livery of the on-board stewards. I love the way they stand by each carriage, with smiles to outclass the cheesiest of air stewards. I love the seats, the loos, the carpet and the wittily designed folding tables.

I love it all. Except – and gosh how it pains me to say it – the food. The food is an absolute fucking disgrace. I'm not often moved to profanity in this column. But when you board the Eurostar, with all its above-mentioned delights, travelling First Class because you're on holiday and you want to treat yourself, and you're on your way to France, the gastronomic Mecca, and your fantasies about *boudins* and *nougatine glacée aux framboises* are starting to hit freefall, you expect at the very least that Eurostar caterers will do something to fuel, not suffocate, your dreams.

Nothing fancy or elaborate is needed; no Michelin star frills are asked for. Just something thoughtful, simple, satisfying – a bit of charcuterie to start with, a little tub of *rillettes*, perhaps, or even just a simple salad of *frisé*, croutons and Gruyère. Something cold would do me for a main course, too – a nice plate of *jambon de Bayonne* with potato salad in a chivey mayonnaise wouldn't be too hard to put together. And if the market research insists that something hot needs to be offered, then how about something that was designed to be reheated? A little bowl of *cassoulet*, for example, or a *petit salé* with lentils?

But what did they offer us? I'll tell you, though it makes me shudder with mounting rage to recall it. Our menu began with something called blue cheese and pear pâté, the French translation of which was *quenelles de fromage bleu et de poires*. Sounds terribly grand, doesn't it? As far as I could tell, this pâté was made by mixing up a mound of Danish Blue (the cheapest, nastiest, blue cheese there is) with a few (almost untraceable in my portion) finely chopped tinned pears, and making it into little rugby-ball shapes with two spoons. Whoever came up with that trick should think about heading back to catering college for another few years (and preferably not the one they just graduated from).

This cynical opener was followed by a choice between turkey and chickpeas. The turkey was dry, colourless, flavourless and, thankfully perhaps, odourless: the kind of which Bernard Matthews (and only he) would have been proud. It came on a bed of 'spring greens' that had lost all their spring and most of their green, having been cooked into a cowpat-coloured sludge.

The chickpea curry, a vegetarian option, at least had the virtue of tasting of something – i.e. curry. But it was a bog-standard concoction of curry spices of the kind one would find in a (very) average provincial high street curry house. It came with overcooked rice, and an equally average vegetable curry.

The dessert was just as devoid of imagination – a purée of apricots and strawberries on top of which sat a Madeleine-like cake. As it had arrived at the same time as the starter, the cake just got soggier and soggier. The flavour of the purée wasn't entirely unpleasant, but it was more or less just baby food.

In the course of sorting out the illustration that accompanies this article my editor found herself talking to Roger, one of the PRs for Eurostar. I'm guessing Roger has had to deal with a number of scathing reviews of the Eurostar food before, because he said, rather defensively, something along the lines of 'I hope Hugh realises we're not trying to compete with top London restaurants. We're just trying to provide a simple meal for our first-class passengers'. Well, I'm afraid that doesn't wash with me. The term First Class implies a certain level of service and quality of product and has done for centuries. If Eurostar does not want to mislead its public, it should rename the service First Class Except For The Food, Which Is Dreadful.

On the other hand I feel extremely sorry for poor Roger. How can you do public relations for a company which is feeding its public such uninteresting garbage?

May 1999

Telling porkies about bacon

We've all had to learn to read between the lines of food labels over the years. These days, any self-respecting consumer knows that, for example, the word 'traditional' actually means 'mass produced by technology developed in the eighties'.

Similarly, most of us now understand that where eggs are concerned the phrase 'farm fresh' is entirely meaningless, unless the word 'farm' calls to mind a stalag of concrete and wire in which chickens are imprisoned in their tens of thousands. And by the same hypocritical token, the conspicuous flagging on a package of the words 'contains no artificial colouring' is pretty much a guarantee that the primary flavours in a product are the work of men in white coats with degrees in chemistry.

One descriptive food word which one might reasonably have considered not merely innocent, but somehow beyond corruption, if only because its meaning is, or ought to be, so unequivocal, is 'crispy'. Yet I have, in the past few weeks, bought a couple of products which demand a whole new definition for this popular foodie epithet. If 'crispy' can now be taken to denote a substance or product that is soft, wet, floppy and capable of being folded into several sections without breaking, then the crispy bacon sandwich on sale aboard Virgin's trains may be taken as the marker for this updated sense of the word.

But it would be unfair to single out Virgin for their work at the cutting edge of modern English usage. Only this morning I discovered that European Rail Catering, who make the sandwiches for a number of the train operating franchises, have adopted a similarly flexible interpretation of the word.

I'm no linguistic conservative, but I can't help feeling that both parties are a little ahead of their time. Might I therefore suggest that, until such time as the respected lexicographers at Oxford and Chambers concur with this latest definition of 'crispy', anyone who encounters a bacon sandwich whose consistency falls clearly within the new parameters follows my example, by slipping the rashers in question into an envelope, and posting them to the chairman of the company responsible for their crispiness, or otherwise.

November 1997

A Moroccan pigeon's revenge

I just took a week's holiday in Morocco. And now I think I know just a little bit about what Hell is really like. Don't get me wrong. Morocco is not at all like Hell. In fact, it's pretty heavenly. But that's the whole point of Hell, isn't it? If it wasn't for the fact that it was so close to being Heaven, the misery wouldn't be half so profound.

We were in the stunning fishing port of Essaouira, where the Atlantic pounds the craggy limestone rocks which form the ramparts of the Medina. Our plan was to do very little except gorge ourselves on the daily catch of sardines, bream, spider crabs and mantis shrimps. We did the sardines on day one – split to make a double fillet, smeared with a stuffing of garlic and coriander and grilled over charcoal. Outstanding.

I had one further mission, to investigate the famous Moroccan *pastilla* – a parcel of wafery pastry filled with an exotic concoction of meat (classically pigeon), almonds, spices, sugar and eggs. I'd done enough research on this dish to work out a pretty respectable version at home, cook it on television and put it in *The River Cottage Cookbook*. But I'd never eaten one in Morocco. My plan was to try as many *pastillas* as possible – and become the finest practitioner of the dish outside of the Arab world. A noble ambition, surely, if a little unrealistic?

I had my first *pastilla* on our first evening. I felt it was good, but not great. The almond, egg and pigeon were in layers, and I felt the balance was tipped too far in favour of the nuts, sugar and spices, at the top. The meat, at the bottom, was a bit lost – and a bit dry.

My next chance came unexpectedly the following day. We had been directed to a rooftop café (by a wood-carver whose advanced understanding of pester power meant our son Oscar was now proudly carrying a three-foot long sculpture of a swordfish under his arm). We drank mint tea and watched the sea crashing on the rocks. We hadn't been planning to eat until later, but when I spotted that the ubiquitous *pastilla* was listed under *Specialités de la maison*, I couldn't resist sneaking one in.

The speed of its arrival should have made me wary. It could hardly have been made to order. Its temperature was also suspect – hottish, but not so as you had to wait before tackling it. None of this worried me, for the simple reason that my *pastilla* – quite a different animal from the one I had eaten the night before – was delicious. The pigeon meat was so tender as to be in shreds. The almonds were mixed through the meat, and the filling was also flecked with leafy green herbs.

The well-proportioned Moroccan lady who had cooked it was friendly and very forthcoming. No, she insisted, there were no eggs in it – that was right for a chicken *pastilla*, not for a pigeon one. (A controversial position, according to my research, but an intriguing one.) Yes, the pigeon was cooked for a very long time. And then the cooking juices were mixed with the almonds, a little sugar and cinnamon. Not just coriander, but another herb too – parsley, I deduced – was the green stuff mixed up with the meat. And she made it yesterday, she said. The flavours had had time to mingle. That was another reason it tasted so good.

That one's definitely going to be a contender, I said to Marie, as we left. And as we stepped on to the street I felt my stomach give a little lurch.

It was about four hours later that the little bug – or the little bugger, as I now tend to think of him – struck. *Giardia lamblia*, I believe, is his name – I read all about him in my *Lonely Planet* guide. Thanks to him I spent most of the next week on the loo. Don't finish this sentence if you're squeamish – but if shitting through the eye of a needle was an Olympic sport, then I would have a gold medal by now.

I didn't eat another *pastilla*. Or any more sardines. And not a bream, or a spider crab, or a mantis shrimp passed my lips. Bananas, bread, and flat Coca Cola were all I could get away with. When I recklessly dared a lentil soup in the square in Marrakech on my last night, I made the loo of a nearby hotel with only seconds to spare.

So the joys of authentic Moroccan pastries are still unknown to me. And the mysterious alchemy of the tagine eludes me still. Oh, I know what they look like. I know what they smell like. I have devoured them greedily in my imagination, over and over again. But all I tasted was a sour smidgin of Hell.

The horrible fate of Tantalus was to wake each morning in Hades with a raging hunger, and a feast fit for the gods laid out before him. But everything he reached out for simply crumbled to dust. If you're still down there, old boy, my heart goes out to you, it really does.

December 2002

Ski cuisine

There are many things to look forward to on a skiing holiday – blizzards, broken legs, barmy bar prices and so on. It's all part of the fun, of course, and if you are incredibly lucky you may even get a few days of sunshine and some decent snow to ski on. What you will almost certainly not get – and what regular ski bums have learnt to live without – is exciting or interesting grub to fuel your energetic exploits on the slopes.

This is surprising, given that the vast majority of skiers take their holidays in France, Italy or Switzerland – countries where they know a thing or two about eating well. Not so surprising, when you realise that in most cases the food is cooked for them by upper middle class English girls who have 'done a course'.

These are the legendary Chalet Girls, who are usually infuriating in three important ways:

1) They ski much better than anyone in your party.

2) You can't get them into bed because they are already knocking off a muscle-bound ski instructor.

3) (This is the rule to which there are the least exceptions.) They barely know how to boil an egg.

They do, however, make a mean white sauce – so floury you could paper walls with it. And what's more, they make it every night. Sometimes it has hardboiled eggs in it, sometimes broccoli – but usually it has tuna. On a really good day you might get all three.

Tinned tuna is the staple ingredient of ski cuisine, a fact onto which the ski resort supermarkets have long ago cottoned. Go to the main supermarket in Val d'Isère, Verbier or Méribel and you will find an entire aisle devoted to tuna. Every evening between six and seven o'clock (prime time shopping in ski resorts) this aisle will be crammed with the rosy-cheeked pearl-and-ponytail brigade filling their trolleys with a hundredweight of Jean Ouest. It's an awesome sight.

Anyone with the temerity to question the repetitive nature of this chalet menu and suggest something a little more *exotique* will get short shrift. 'Have you any idea how expensive fresh vegetables/mince/chicken/bacon/horse (delete as appropriate) is up here?' The problem is, with most tour operators you have paid in advance for your food, and the chalet girls have a limited – extremely limited – budget with which to cater for your party. So you've only brought enough money to buy booze for the chalet and lunch every day at the on-piste restaurant, where a plate of chips costs 55 francs and Coke's a snip if you can get it for 30. You'd like to fork out the extra tenner a head for a plate of grilled horse but you're all flat broke.

Your only relief is the chalet girl's night off. She gets taken out to the ski resort's most expensive restaurant to eat lobster, foie gras and *magret de canard* with Bruno or Klaus, or Jean Baptiste. Your party goes out for a cheese fondue.

A cookery book has been brought to my attention which wholeheartedly confirms my prejudices about ski-resort cookery. *The Bladon Lines Chalet Girl Cookery Book* is a selection of recipes from 'the experts in glamorous cooking on a small budget'. The prime motivation of chalet girls is confirmed as early as the foreword: 'Any chalet girl worth her salt will be a keen skier and she'll want to spend the maximum number of hours out of the chalets and on the mountainside . . . our girls . . . become experts in knocking up a stunning male in a couple of hours.' Well, all right, it says 'meal', but I'm sure it's a misprint.

True to this ideal, the book has some of the most effortless recipes I have ever seen in print. The instructions for a dish called *noodles haute Nendaz* would not bear a lot of editing: 'Mix all the ingredients together and serve'. Verbose by comparison is *salade al dente*: 'Mix the vinaigrette with the mayonnaise and toss with the prepared vegetables.'

The book is interspersed with priceless 'chalet girl comments and economy tips' such as 'This is an excellent way of using up meringues that have gone wrong' or 'Put all dregs of wine in a sealed bottle for cooking'. Glaring omissions of chalet girl thrift presumably include 'Pour tapwater into recycled mineral water bottles and take the difference out of your shopping budget', and 'Collect cigarette butts from the ash-trays to make your own rollups'. I guess these could be saved for the next edition . . .

February 1992

Suffering helplessly at the hands of incompetent cooks is a misery, but a more
refined irritation is being told that one cannot have what one wants in the first
place. And it's particularly galling to be denied a treat, not because the chef
can't do it, but because the government won't let him . . .

Brainless

'I'm sorry, we don't have any brains' – not an excuse for slow
service from a waitress at the Fashion Café, but a tragic announcement from the proprietor of my favourite Middle Eastern
restaurant, Istanbul Iskembecisi, on Stoke Newington Road. This
establishment has always specialised in serving dishes made from
the parts of a sheep that other chefs dare not reach for. Their
lamb's brain croquettes, served with *kiri*, a delicious salad of
cracked wheat, chopped peppers, tomatoes, garlic and parsley,
was one of my favourite dishes on any menu in London. Now,
apparently, they just can't get the brains.

I called MAFF who confirmed that, under the grimly named
'Heads of Goats and Sheep Order, 1996' it is now illegal to offer
sheep's brains for sale as food. This was perhaps understandable
in the case of cow's brains (banned over two years ago), if only
as a temporary response to public fears about BSE. But sheep
offal has never been associated with the disease in humans, and
MAFF are unable to offer any scientific basis for the ban
whatsoever. Most sheep are still fed on a natural diet of grass,
and the fact is that it has been illegal to feed sheep on any animal
offal for over two years. Is this no longer considered the
guarantee of safety it once was? MAFF couldn't help me on
that one. Clearly I am going to have to graze sheep in my
window box and slaughter them myself.

I would, too, because I love brains. The creamy, curdy texture
and mild flavour are inimitable by any other body part. They have
long been a vital ingredient in Middle Eastern cooking, and many
Lebanese and Turkish restaurants in London have made their
regular customers very happy over the years by offering them on
their menu. What gives the government the right to remove this

extremely fine delicacy from the London food scene? MAFF wouldn't give me an answer. Could it be, 'I'm sorry, we don't have any brains'?

May 1997

Spineless

The beef on the bone débâcle was thrown into tragicomic relief for me last week when, the day after the ban came into force, I went for dinner at the Grill Room of the Connaught. We were perusing the great and historic menu of this near unfaultable dining room, preserved in aspic since the thirties, when our waiter arrived beside our table with his trolley, or 'chariot' as it is most properly called, on top of which was one of those enormous swivelling silver domes.

'The roast this evening', he announced, 'is a whole sirloin of beef.' And he swivelled his dome to reveal a fillet of meat which, while it might have looked pretty fine on the sideboard of your average domestic dining room, looked more like a lost sausage in the middle of the vast desert of its silver platter.

'Tonight', he announced, with an expression of pained professionalism, like an out of work actor who is doing children's parties dressed as a clown, 'we are serving it *off the bone.*' It was the 'Tonight' that got me, pronounced with a heavy emphasis that implied he hoped this was just a temporary aberration – as if tomorrow he might wake up from this nightmare and find himself returned to the proper order of things, where the Connaught's whole roast sirloin comes magnificently, as it always has, with chine and ribs intact.

I passed on the sirloin, and ordered a roast woodcock instead. It came on the bone, pink and bloody, with the frazzled head and neck on the side. The head was split, as is the ancient custom, to reveal the brains, which are a delicacy. Here is some consolation for customers and kitchens bullied by a busybody government. The Connaught may be struggling to come to terms with the indignity of serving beef off the bone, but they should be justly proud to be probably the last restaurant in London serving brains of any kind.

December 1997

Among the hardest things to swallow, I have always found, are the medicines intended for over-indulgence. That's the catch 22 of the hangover.

Does the hair of your dog bite?

P. G. Wodehouse, in one of his Mulliner stories, lists six different symptoms of hangover which may afflict the sufferer in varying combinations: the Atomic, the Broken Compass, the Cement Mixer, the Comet, the Gremlin Boogie and the Sewing Machine. This is the time of year when all six versions, like the unwanted relatives you may share them with, come to plague you at once, and for a period of several days. What can you possibly do?

Surprisingly, the medical description of the hangover squares up rather neatly with Wodehouse's account though the terminology shows a lot less empathy with the sufferer. 'The hangover is a multisystem syndrome,' explains Eric Beck, consultant physician at the North London Hospital. 'Regular symptoms include headache, nausea, vertigo, dehydration, depression and oversensitivity to light and noise.' This last problem, which I am inclined to equate with Wodehouse's Gremlin Boogie, once prompted a letter to the manufacturers of one favourite hangover treatment: 'Dear Alka Seltzer, please could you make your tablets quieter.'

But, as with the next most frequent national ailment, the common cold, the medical fraternity offers little prospect of a cure for hangovers. The best it can recommend is 'symptomatic treatment'.

'The headache', explains Beck, 'is best treated with a gastric, non-irritant analgesic, such as paracetamol. Fluid replacement is also helpful and, in severe cases, sugar replacement with glucose-added drinks. Apart from that, I can only recommend withdrawal to a darkened, silent room and further sleep, which should help to facilitate a natural recovery.'

If conventional medicine is fairly clear on the sensible approach to the blinder behind the eyes, there is no shortage of self-styled amateur witch-doctors, most of them regular sufferers themselves, to offer you a more miraculous alternative. This usually takes the form of some magic pick-me-up, 'guaranteed' to restore you to peak condition in a matter of minutes.

But in every case 'pick-me-up' is a feeble euphemism for 'cocktail'. The Prairie Oysters, Bloody Marys, bullshots and nogs that you are likely to be offered on Boxing or New Year's Day by a co-suffering host all rely on the dubious 'hair of the dog principle' and ignore the more reliable, but less cited, drinker's maxim that 'whoever got high, must come down'.

Accepting the inevitability of the 'downer' is the key to tackling a hangover successfully; the whole concept of a cure is bursting with false hope. Treatment must therefore be aimed at distracting or comforting the sufferer.

Having sex usually has both of these effects and often promotes a restorative post-coital sleep. It is not an option for everybody, though. Idle telly-watching is a less athletic alternative, though it can challenge one of the symptoms – oversensitivity to light and sound – just a little too fiercely.

Some patented hangover cures, unwittingly perhaps, successfully exploit the distraction tactic, others the comfort. There is a fearsome product called Dr Harris's Original Pick-me-up. This is a pink liquid whose sinus-ripping reek suggests that one of its principal ingredients is ammonia. Those brave enough to take an occasional sip will certainly find themselves thinking less about their hangover and more about the cruelty of a mind that could devise quite such a foul-tasting formula. One celebrity tippler, at least, believes that the concoction is cruel only to be kind: Harris's Pick-me-up bears the Royal Warrant of Queen Elizabeth the Queen Mother.

A health food shop is perhaps an unlikely port of call for a hardened sufferer of hangovers, but it is one that can definitely afford some relief for the afflicted. *Ume-sho bancha* is a Japanese restorative made from soya extract, fermented Ume plums and a concentrate of *kukicha* (twig tea). It may not have mystical oriental powers, but it makes a warming and palatable brew, and is a comforting way to replace lost fluids, salts and minerals.

More indulgent still is a flirtation with aromatherapy. Essential oils of basil, grapefruit, juniper and rosemary are recommended – one drop each in a hot bath. Better still, a distraction as well as a comfort would be a massage with a vegetable oil impregnated with two drops of each of the essential oils. The problem is finding someone competent, willing and less hungover than you, to administer the treatment.

There is one treatment for a hangover that would, I am confident, be a genuine cure, if it were ever possible to perform it. If only I could flip off the top of my head, remove my brain, and place it in a bucket of fizzing Alka Seltzer for half an hour, then pop it back in and replace the lid, I'm sure I would feel much better.

December 1992

And finally in this section, a confessional. I know it comes easily to me to work up a bit of righteous indignation when I see what some in the food business – the multiple food retailers and industrial food giants, mainly – are doing to our land, our livestock, and our food culture. But I hope I'm not too self-righteous to recognise, on occasion, my own shortcomings . . .

Confessions of a serial plate picker

I would like to make a public apology. More than that, I would like to announce, for the record, that I truly intend to mend my ways. It seems I have, for some time (a couple of decades, at least), been regularly offending my family, my friends and my work colleagues at mealtimes. I am finally facing up to the fact that I have a problem: I am a habitual food thief – a serial stealer of tempting morsels on other people's plates. I now realise – and it has taken me a pitifully long time to draw this conclusion – that it is wrong, and it has to stop.

But I know it will be hard. The compulsion to snaffle the last piece of crispy duck (for example) on my neighbour's plate is over-powering, even, or perhaps especially, when I know he or she has been saving it for the end (precisely because it is such a fine morsel). Sometimes I barely even know I have done it. Exchanges like the following are not uncommon:

'I can't believe you just did that!'

'Did what?'

'Took that strawberry off my plate. The one with the small but perfectly sized blob of cream on it. The one I'd been saving to the end...'

'I didn't!'

'You did. I just watched you. I was so shocked I couldn't say anything until it was too late...'

'I really don't think it was me. Are you sure you didn't just finish it off subconsciously, while you were listening to your other neighbour's fascinating story?'

'Look. You had the chocolate roulade, right?'

'Yes.'

'So how exactly do you explain that little red streaked smear of cream on the end of your fork?...'

I know that I am not a lone perpetrator of this crime. I suspect my fellow offenders are mostly, but not exclusively, men. We have a greater gift for self-delusion than women. And in this case the delusion is a mighty one. We kid ourselves that there is some playful charm, a forgivable, even lovable quality about our behaviour. We even seem to think these acts of petty gastronomic theft bestow and elicit affection on and from our victims, so that our plate-picking habit actually makes a positive contribution to the general *bonhomie* of a shared dining experience.

In fact, a common defence which I have been known to employ goes like this: 'It's not stealing, it's sharing. Er... try a bit of mine...' (To which the likely reply will be, 'Why exactly would I want a withered lettuce leaf with a yellowy brown bit on the edge? You never even offered me a scrap of one of your scallops, and now they're all gone!')

These scenarios are most often acted out with a female fellow diner – not infrequently my wife, and sometimes even my mother (the shame!). For although this is not straightforwardly a battle of the sexes (I have stolen plenty of fine things from the plates of men and boys) it is certainly compounded by the general tendency of men to eat all the most tempting looking things on their plates first, while women so often save the best until last.

Whoever my victims are, such behaviour rarely passes without comment. And I have hardly ever met anyone who didn't mind, at least a bit, having their plate picked. Given that such mealtime skirmishes have been going on as long as I can remember, on an almost daily basis, you may be wondering how it is possible that I have taken so long to achieve any insight into the severity of my problem, and the extent of the accumulated irritation and misery I have caused.

The reason is, I believe, that I, and others like me, am afforded the powerful protection of the tacit social rituals of eating. In each individual case, the damage is relatively small (I don't eat all the food on their plate – just the bit they wanted the most). And so they are constrained to keep the irritation expressed relatively mild. However annoyed they may be, nobody wants to make too much of a fuss over a little bit of food, lest it be thought it is them, and not me, who has a problem with their food, and is allowing it to spoil the party.

So, inevitably, it has taken a bit of a shock to bring me to my senses. As so often in life, to bring about change, one bold individual must speak out, and give voice to the thoughts that many have merely internalised for so long.

That individual is a cameraman with whom I have been working regularly for almost ten years. I am very fond of him, despite the fact that he gives me a consistently hard time, in an imaginatively foul-mouthed way, whenever we work together. We must have sat at the same table dozens if not hundreds of times. Which means the amount of food I have had off his plate over the years could probably be measured in kilos. I've taken a barrage of abuse as a result – but never so much that I wasn't able to persuade myself, if I thought about it at all, that it was all good fun.

That all changed last week, during a very excellent dinner at the

Star Inn at Harome, Yorkshire, near where we had been filming. He was enjoying his slow roast belly of pork, with a particularly provocative pile of fine crackling on the side. I went for what was probably the penultimate piece with my thumb and forefinger. For once he was too quick for me, and gave me a sharp jab with his fork. 'No!' he said. 'You are not fucking having it! And if you do that to me one more time, I swear I will pick up my fucking fork and stab your hand so fucking hard I will pin it to the fucking table! And I mean that!' The rest of the table was reduced to awed silence. And I could tell they approved his sentiments.

The severity of this threat was eased somewhat by the twinkle in his eye, and the fact that we were well into our third pints. I do not believe he is truly a violent man, or that he would ever really have carried out his threat. In fact, it was not so much the colourful language, or the graphic, *Goodfellas*-style punishment he was conjuring, that shook me up so much. It was a subtle nuance of his grammar: '. . . if you do that to me one more time . . .'

Those words shattered the biggest delusion of all: that mine is a mischief perpetrated not on a person, but on a plate of food. And therefore, that no harm is really done, that this is a victimless crime.

I now know differently. I have discussed it with other recurrent targets of my greed – and they're all on his side. They have collectively encouraged me to confront my disorder. They have promised to act swiftly and ruthlessly if ever they see my fork or my finger hovering towards their plate. The suffering, they say, has gone on too long.

Now it will be my turn to suffer – the twisted agony of self-denial. It will be hard, and it will be painful. But it will be no more than I deserve.

November 2005

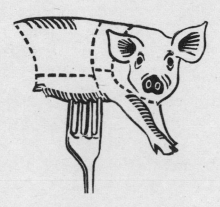

I Don't Mind if I Do

Expanding my culinary horizons,
at home and abroad

Here we journey into the more unusual – and often inspiring – foods that I have encountered on my travels, both at home and abroad. Incidentally, the one notable update on the following article would be the transfer of the entry on 'bat' from the section headed 'Still on the wish list' to 'Been there, scoffed that'. This piece also contains the first acknowledgement of the moniker that has become the title of this book.

Taste not, want not

It has been said that I will eat anything. This is, of course, nonsense. Medium Density Fibreboard soaked in paraffin served between two discs of foam rubber has never got me salivating (which is why I steer clear of McDonald's), and a fried egg that still has a pool of runny egg white clinging to the yolk is a definite no-no.

Still, I must admit that it was with some pride that I read, in one review of my series *A Cook on the Wild Side*, that I had been given the sobriquet 'Hugh Fearlessly Eatsitall'. I was less pleased with another critic who previewed the show by saying 'Hairy Hugh dredges up more muck from the canal for his grubby cooking pot.' Had the critic in question been able to join me in my repast of zander grilled on fennel seeds with wild juniper sauce, I'm confident he would not have been so scathing. Although perhaps he is more at home with the aforementioned fast food.

The truth is, if I may be modest for a moment, that there was not a meal I cooked in my two series that did not have some genuine culinary merit – even if it might not have been to the taste of all-comers. (I will acknowledge that fried sand eels – mushy texture and bland in the extreme – are a possible exception. But I would never have tried them, had I not failed to catch a sea bass – that king of fish, for which the unfortunate sand eels were intended merely as bait.)

I would always defend my palate as adventurous, not undiscerning.

After all, I like my hogweed shoots strictly al dente and my impala liver pink, but not too bloody. I will willingly admit, however, to taking some pleasure in tasting foods that others shun, or that few get the chance to get their gobs around. Some might regard this as a childish form of foodie train spotting – or an oral fixation bordering on the perverse. But it seems to me obvious that anything that is regarded as good food by some nation or tribe on the planet, must at least have the potential to please me too – provided I can free myself from western cultural constraints. Consequently, my motto is: 'Taste everything once – except fat-free cakes and anything made by Bernard Matthews.'

I have applied this omnivorous maxim to fruit and vegetables, as much as to protein. But I cannot deny that the thrill of sampling something new is often that much greater when it is something that has run, swum, flown or crawled. I don't quite know why this is: perhaps my genetic make up is simply more hunter than gatherer. Anyway, the result is that I have enjoyed many magical mouthfuls over the years, and made treats of some curious creatures, as well as the anatomical details of the more familiar farm animals. This magazine has asked me to share them with you and it is my pleasure to do so. I shall also describe, in anticipation of future feasts, just a few of the many arcane beasts celebrated for their delicacy in whatever part of the world they happen to occur, which I have yet to enjoy the privilege of tasting. If anyone has samples to send me, I'll happily take them. But no Golden Drummers, please.

Incidentally, I make no apology for the absence in my guide of such alleged aphrodisiacs as tiger's penis, walrus's testicles, and rhino's horn – and not only because their culinary potential is at least as questionable as any alleged physiological effect. Even a super-omnivore such as myself has principles – and I happen to believe those particular organs have a far more vital role to play in the propagation of little tigers and walruses than in increasing the reproductive ambitions (though surely not the performance) of the kind of egotistical maniacs who should probably not be allowed to have children anyway.

A further word to those surprised by the omission of ostrich, kangaroo and crocodile from my list: come off it! In these sad days of gimmicky gastronomy, you can find these poor products of neo-agriculture on the menu in the average suburban steak house. Catch a wild one yourself, on the other hand, and you may have a story.

1: Favourite body parts

Brains

Their unique creamy texture, contained within a lovely crispy surface that can be achieved by shallow or deep frying, make brains truly one of my favourite foods. I first tasted calf's brains almost ten years ago at the River Cafe, where I worked as a sous chef. They used to be a regular on the menu there, tossed in flour and fried up with crispy sage leaves and salted capers. Sadly, the sale of brains has now been banned by MAFF, in the wake of the BSE scare: an understandable measure, perhaps, in the case of calf's brains, but ludicrous as far as sheep is concerned – given the assurances we have had from MAFF itself that sheep offal constitutes no risk to human consumers. I live in the hope that the ban may soon be lifted, and in the meantime satisfy my desire on occasional trips to France, where brains are still widely available in butchers.

Lamb's testicles

In terms of texture, testicles are not dissimilar to brains. When well prepared (they need to be marinated in salt water or lemon juice), the taste is mild and pleasant, but they can have a tendency to kidney-like bitterness. If you've got the balls to try them, the place to go is Al-Basha, a Lebanese restaurant on Kensington High Street.

Cow's udders

A delicacy I have only once encountered on a menu – in a Korean restaurant in Tokyo. They have a mild taste and a chewy texture, a little like tripe, but come up nice and crispy when cooked in thin strips on a charcoal grill.

Pig's ears and tails

La queue et l'oreille (the tail and the ear) is a Parisian brasserie classic. The place to try it is the fantastically glamorous fin de siècle dining room of La Coupole in Paris. After a lengthy simmering to tenderise the skin, the hand-sized ear and foot-long tail are crisped up under a hot salamander, and served with tartare sauce. Outstanding.

Rook's breast

I have never seen rooks on sale in any shop, so this is definitely a do-it-yourself delicacy. Young rooks are quite palatable until mid-July (after that they become tough and sinewy), but they are best of all just after leaving the nest (mid-May to June). Known as 'branchers' they are quite easy to shoot at this time, provided you are skilled with a .22 rifle or air rifle. A shotgun will make mincemeat of them. Fry the little breasts in olive oil, and deglaze the pan juices with a little wine or vinegar to make a sauce.

Squirrel's haunch

'Fury as TV chef cooks Tufty!' ran a headline in one newspaper, when I cooked the meaty back legs of a couple of grey squirrels in the New Forest episode of my series. Yet the Forestry Commission kills thousands of squirrels by trapping and poisoning each year (they do untold damage to young trees). Under the circumstances, it's a criminal waste not to eat them, and I refuse to be put off by those brandishing the fluffy tail factor. They are better than rabbit, and as tender and flavoursome as the best game birds (I know one New Forest chef who cheekily puts squirrel on the menu as 'flightless partridge').

Donkey salami

I like donkeys when they are alive, and they are one of those creatures (along with dogs) for whom the working relationship between man and beast produces feelings of uncase in me — along with most of the rest of my compatriots — about consuming them. But when I came across a market stall in the Charente region of France selling home-made donkey salami, curiosity got the better of me. I tried it, and it was very, very good. I found some consolation in the fact that the woman at the stall who sold and made the salami assured me that her donkeys led happy working lives. She had an open honesty about her that convinced me she was speaking the truth.

2: Wildlife of the African plain

After I left university I travelled around Southern Africa for six months, researching a paper for the Endangered Wildlife Trust. You will gather from this section that I do not subscribe to the sentimentalist's view that looking at wild animals and eating them are mutually exclusive pleasures. Wildlife is a resource that has to be managed sustainably, to bring maximum benefit to the African people who are its guardians. And a sustainable harvest of wild meat is something western conservationists must learn to respect.

Giraffe

Properly prepared, and cooked rare, giraffe's meat steak can be better than steak or venison. The meat has a natural sweetness that may not be to everybody's taste, but is certainly to mine when grilled over an open fire. The famous Nairobi restaurant Carnivores, which serves all manner of African game, does superb spit roast haunch of giraffe, an impressively huge cut of meat that they will carve for you at the table.

Warthog

In Swaziland I helped cook a special lunch for Prince Rupert of the Netherlands, who came to visit a new rhino reserve there. The centrepiece was a young warthog, which had been marinated for three days in a mixture of wine, peanut oil – and Bovril! My job was to keep the beast basted during a long slow roast over hot coals. I'm pleased, if not modest, to report that it produced the best crackling I have ever tasted. The meat was pretty good too.

Impala

When someone asks me what is the best thing I have ever eaten, I am prepared to risk accusations of being deeply pretentious to tell them about the time I sat around a bush fire in the Luangwa valley, Zambia, grilling little cubes of liver from a freshly killed impala on the end of a twig.

Kudu

This large antelope, with its magnificent spiralling antlers, is regarded as a little on the tough side to be cooked quick and served pink. But it makes superb biltong: strips of the meat are rubbed with salt and spices, and hung in the sun to dry. The resulting product, a bit like a lean salami without a skin, is cut into short lengths which can be kept in the pocket. A bit of biltong and a cold beer, when the sun goes down, is one of the greatest pleasures of the African safari.

3: Creepy crawlies I have known

I am quite prepared to admit that for me, eating insects is largely a matter of bravado. I have yet to try any about which I would be remotely tempted to use the word 'delicious'. On the other hand, I always like to remind people that some of our most delectable seafood (prawns, shrimps, lobsters and crabs) are really just aquatic insects – so I think I should at least remain open to offers.

Maggots

I once produced a film about an Essex entrepreneur, Bruce Silcock, and his plans to build the world's largest maggot farm. His industry exists to feed the angler's insatiable appetite for live maggots as bait. But Bruce was convinced that maggots had potential far beyond that. He claimed that maggots, once separated from the decaying meat they feed on, were a clean and highly nutritious source of protein, with potential for development into products not just for animals, but even for human consumption.

To prove the point, he put half a pint of wriggling larvae into a blender and flicked the switch. The resulting gunge was tipped into a hot frying pan, and stirred into a kind of scrambled omelette. Bruce ate forkfuls of the stuff with confidence, and no apparent distaste. It seemed an appropriate gesture of solidarity with a man who had given us so much of his time to have a little nibble. I won't say they were good, but it was a big enough surprise to discover that they did not actually taste foul. I haven't spoken to Bruce for a while, but if things have gone according to plan, the first maggot-burgers should be rolling off the production line pretty soon.

Woodlice

The woodlouse ought to have culinary potential, if only because it is such a close relative of one of my favourite foods, the shrimp. I put this theory to the test in the last series of *A Cook on the Wild Side*, with the help of some eager young grub-gatherers – three young kids who were staying on a neighbouring barge. They provided me with some fine, fat specimens, which I cooked for barely a minute in plenty of boiling water. I tasted them in this state and was delighted to find they really did taste a bit like shrimps, albeit with a slightly bosky note offsetting the fishy sweetness. The only drawback is an overly high ratio of shell to meat – even a big woodlouse is too small to peel. The solution, I felt, was to turn them into fritters, which I made up from a lentil purée with a bit of chopped wild garlic as an extra flavouring. The resulting 'woodlice bhajis' were pretty good, with the distribution of woodlice through the batter adding a pleasant crunch. In all, it must rate as the pinnacle of my culinary experiments with insects to date – though I can't help feeling there must be heights left to scale.

4: Sexy seafood

Most of the following sea-dwellers are alleged aphrodisiacs. Not all of them worked for me, but all make pretty interesting eating nonetheless.

Chitons

The chiton, which clings to rocks with twice the tenacity of a limpet, looks like a small armadillo without any legs. But beneath its articulated shell is a bright orange morsel of meat, which is rightly savoured by those prepared to take the trouble to prise it from its perch (a flexible fine-bladed knife is the best tool for the job). I have encountered it in the greatest profusion on the coast of Kenya and all over the Seychelles, but it occurs in various sub-species all over the tropics. I have on several occasions gathered a starter-sized portion of these molluscs. The meat can be removed from the shell, boiled until tender (around 30 minutes), and then tossed in garlic butter. Or, for a more instant snack, they can be cooked in their shells in the embers of a beach fire.

Fugu

The fugu is legendary in Japanese culinary culture, and the southern port of Shimonoseki, where the largest catch is landed, has adopted the fish as its municipal mascot. What makes it interesting, from a culinary point of view, is that it is deadly poisonous. However, so highly regarded is its flesh (served raw with a pungent soy-based dipping sauce) that chefs are prepared to undergo a seven-year apprenticeship to learn the meticulous art of preparing the meat so as to reduce the risk to an absolute minimum.

It's hard to say whether fugu deserves the high esteem lavished on it by enthusiasts. I have eaten it several times, and it certainly makes palatable enough *sashimi*: a pleasant flavour is combined with a very firm texture, which allows the fish to be sliced into transparently thin slices. What makes it really special, however, is the elaborate ritual that has evolved to honour the fish (and thereby the diner) whenever it is served: a fugu dinner can comprise up to nine courses besides the *sashimi*, including a soup made from the bones, deep-fried fillets of baby fugu, *sake* infused with fugu fins, and crispy nibbles of fried fugu skin. Add to that the thrill that no doubt derives from the perceived risk (a small number of people still die every year from fugu poisoning, though almost invariably when they have tried to prepare the fish themselves), and you may or may not begin to understand why people will pay enormous prices to play this time-honoured game of *poisson roulette*.

Goose barnacles

These fist-sized shellfish proliferate on the wild west coast of South America, especially Chile, where they are rightly regarded as among the finest fruits of the sea. The flavour is very like crab, and sucking out the strands of white meat from the crusty brown shell is not unlike dealing with a hefty crab claw – a challenge that repays every calorie of effort.

Sea urchins

The spiny urchin is well protected from predators, but enthusiastic gastronomes have found ways to breach this barrier to get at the fleshy orange corals (known as 'tongues') within. A special gadget called a *coupe oursin*, which I covet but do not yet own, has been devised to perform this task, but all you really need is a glove and a good pair of scissors. The taste is sweet, with a slight and not unpleasant note of iodine, which derives from the urchin's diet of kelp and other seaweeds. I have never given much credence to theories of shellfish having aphrodisiac properties, but I once ate 30 sea urchins at a sitting, and at the end of that session I was certainly ready to party.

Sea urchins that are anything less than completely fresh (i.e. alive) are quite unpalatable. I once had a bad urchin in Chile, and it was without doubt the most disgusting thing I have ever put in my mouth.

5: Still on the wish list

There must be literally thousands of creatures, be they mammal, fish, bird or invertebrate, that have at some time been eaten by hungry and hopeful humans. Here are a few that I haven't yet tried, but whose alleged gastronomic potential is certainly intriguing. Perhaps they will be the subjects of future feats.

Armadillo

Armadillo is commonly eaten in South America, and locally popular in Texas, where it is quaintly known as 'possum on the half-shell'.

Badger

Badger is said to make excellent ham. I would never deliberately kill a badger, as the treat of simply seeing one is something I have enjoyed all too rarely. But if ever I encounter a fresh roadkill, I would be tempted to give it a whirl.

Bat

Curried fruit bat is considered a great delicacy in the Seychelles, and it is a matter of some regret that I have been twice to these islands and still not managed to sample it. (It is seasonal, and I have always been there at the wrong time.) However, I am hoping to put this right next time, as a Seychellois friend has promised to put some in the deep freeze for me.

Chinchillas

These are said to be excellent, and, I imagine, similar to squirrel. Chinchillas can be bought alive in this country – but even I draw the line at buying my meat in pet shops.

Dormouse

This shy species of tree-dwelling rodent, almost the size of a squirrel, is said to give excellent meat. It is under threat in this country, so it's not something I would actively pursue. Given its arboreal habits, a roadkill hardly seems on the cards either, so it's probably destined to remain the subject of idle speculation.

Muskrat

This large semi-aquatic rodent, native to North America, has established itself on the continent, and very locally in this country, as a feral descendant of fur farm escapees. I met a French farmer who said he had shot and eaten one, and that it was very good. Some time after, I saw one swimming across a pond in France where I was fishing. I rather optimistically lobbed a rock at it: had I had a better aim, I might have been able to tell you more.

Palolo worm

This is a marine worm that inhabits the coral reefs of the South Pacific. It is collected not for its flesh, but for its eggs, which are cast off in swollen egg sacs in huge quantities every November. Worm caviar is one of the most intriguing culinary concepts I have ever encountered, and I sincerely hope to get the chance to sample it.

Snake

Many species of snake are edible, and on my African travels I was more than ready to give it a go. I almost got my chance when I accidentally ran over a large puff adder, but a secretary bird, who I suspect already had the snake in its sights, made off with it before I could retrieve it.

September 1998

If it swims or flies, eat it

Until last night, I hadn't eaten meat for three weeks. Actually that's not strictly true. I had eaten the flesh of fish, and of cephalopods, and crustacea, and bivalves. It is all meat, of course, in the dictionary definition sense of the word (we say 'there's a lot of meat on this crab', but never 'there's a lot of fish on this trout') – just not in the conventional culinary categories sense of the word. It's an understandable convention, I guess, given that we are ourselves land-dwellers, who innately regard the sea as hostile territory – somewhere to plunder as our ingenuity allows, but not to linger too long. But it irritates me when the fish/meat distinction is dragged into the ethical sphere, as it occasionally is by those who eat fish, but not 'meat', on supposedly moral grounds: 'Let's kill it and eat it if it swims in water but not if it walks on land. And we'll worry about amphibians after dinner.' It's not sharp thinking, in my view.

I digress. I've been on holiday with my family in the Seychelles. Kind of a treat for finishing my latest book. Which, as it happens, is about Meat – in more or less the conventional culinary category sense of the word. (The plan is not to change the linguistic habit of the past several millennia – just to change the shopping, eating and cooking habits of everyone in Britain, and hence the way our meat is produced. And that's the blatant – though by no means irrelevant – plug taken care of.)

Anyway, having immersed myself thoroughly in meat for pretty much the last four years, we left our sheep, cows and a litter of 11 piglets, in the capable hands of my cousin Simon and our part-time stockman Bernie. And we left behind our three beloved freezers – called pork, beef and lamb. And we headed off for the fish-rich waters of these stunning Indian Ocean islands to immerse ourselves instead in the absence of responsibility – and in fish (including cephalopods, crustacea, etc.).

I could crudely summarise the pattern of most days of our holiday thus: in the morning we would generally look at fish – through the lenses (in my case prescription) of our diving masks. In the afternoon we would generally try and catch some fish. And in the evening, as well as at lunchtime, we would invariably eat some fish. Sometimes we would vary things a bit by fishing in the morning, and snorkelling in the afternoon.

And once I went snorkelling after dinner, with an underwater torch to light the coral reef. I managed to pluck an enormous spiny lobster from the seabed. It was remarkably compliant, seeming to come willingly, until I got it back to the surface. Then it flapped its muscly tail with such power and rage that it cut my thumb and I dropped it. It was perhaps just as well. I found out the next day that Seychellois lobsters are currently enjoying the benefit of a closed season, as a conservation measure. It would have been a memorable feast, but technically one for which I could have done time.

It may seem odd to some that one would first want to look at fish as a fascinated and beguiled amateur natural historian, then set all one's cunning and predatory instincts to catching and killing them, next exercise all one's creative powers in the kitchen to make them aromatic and savoury, and finally satisfy one's base hunger by devouring them. But that, in a way, is what it is to be a human being: an aesthete and yet still a savage, a problem-solving intellect shackled to a range of base instincts, a moral being with a brute's appetite.

Not that the 'fish only' thing was any kind of resolution, either ethical or aesthetic. It was just about choosing the best, freshest, most local and delicious 'meat' available on the island. And that, for fairly obvious reasons, was almost entirely coming from the sea. Had the opportunity to eat meat (in the conventional, mammalian, land-based sense of the word), of sound and interesting provenance, presented itself earlier, we would have taken it gladly.

Yet there was an element of unwitting virtue arising from this diet. A diet based on fresh fruit, fish and rice, is pretty sound. You can even add in a generous allowance of beer and rum, and it still looks after you pretty well. Remove the biggest single cause of indigestion – stress. Add in sunshine. Here you have an outstanding recipe for physical and mental recuperation.

The seafood diet finally came to an end yesterday night – the last of our holiday – but with a 'meat' that is hardly conventional, and scarcely land-based either (though it is certainly a mammal). The provenance is excellent. These animals have fed only on the finest, tropical fruits (mangoes and breadfruit are their favourites). They have lived wild and free. And, as with the fish, we had been admiring them throughout our holiday, as they appeared reliably every evening and swooped about in the tropical gloaming.

They are in plentiful supply – so much so that they are regarded as an agricultural pest (and for me that always adds an element of satisfaction to the consumption of a wild meat). They are the reason, in fact, that you can't buy a decent ripe mango in the market. In the old days, they used to shoot them, but since the 1972 coup, there are no guns allowed on the island. Now they are caught in nets, which isn't nearly as efficient, but keeps the meat in far better nick.

This local speciality was prepared for us, by a Seychellois friend of our host, who marinated the meat in lime, garlic and cinnamon leaves and braised it to a subtly spicy sweet-and-sour perfection. And I enjoyed every surprisingly meaty mouthful of it. If you ever get to the Seychelles – and I hope you will – don't pass up the opportunity to sample a curried bat. It's even better than squirrel, and that's high praise indeed.

April 2004

Toasting Tufty

My copy of *Larousse Gastronomique* jumps straight from 'squill-fish' to 'stabilising agent' – which just goes to show that the French do not know everything about food. The missing entry is, of course, 'squirrel'. (I looked under 'grey squirrel', but again there is a glaring omission – between '*grenobloise*' and '*gribiche*'). Happily, where the *Larousse* leaves off, Prue Coats, of Tower Hill Farm in the pretty Hampshire village of Dummer, takes over.

Prue is the widow of the late Archie Coats, legendary pigeon-shooter and one of the most famous countrymen of his generation. In their touching and devoted partnership of more than 35 years, Archie brought into their ample game larder all manner of feathered and furred game – and Prue learned, by force of necessity, to process it, market it and above all, to cook it.

Squirrel is one of Prue's more recent pot adventures – along with rook pie and stuffed carp. Preparations for these, and more traditional gamey fare, are chronicled in her book, *The Poacher's Cookbook*. On a perfectly terrible autumn day last week, I was the recipient of Prue's famously cloud-dispersing hospitality – and squirrel was on the menu.

'People think the idea of eating squirrel is a bit nasty,' said Prue as she tossed the dainty portions of pale pink meat into seasoned flour, 'but when you think about their diet of nuts and berries and things, it's just what's needed to make good, tasty meat. These two are both very young, so they should be quite tender.' The squirrels were due for the speediest of sautées in Prue's wok, so before she did them we sat down to a glass of fine Burgundy and a starter of Prue's superb smoked pigeon pâté. As I munched toast-loads of this rich, lightly smoky paste, cunningly spiked with ginger and vermouth, Prue told me one of her favourite poaching stories.

'Early one morning,' began Prue with a twinkle, 'our farmer friend who owned the land which Archie used to shoot over, came to the door, and announced with an ill-concealed grin: "You've been poached." He had found a beaten-up Daihatsu in the middle of one of his fields, with a boot full of still warm rabbits. So I said rather crossly: "Well, what do you expect me to do about it?" And he said, "Nothing. I've already dealt with it." He'd fetched his JCB and dug a large hole in the ground, and buried the Daihatsu. The next day these two rather worried-looking rough cuts were wandering around asking "Anybody seen our car?"'

In other tales the poacher fares rather better than the gamekeeper. For example, the cocky poacher who used to bait gamekeepers by hanging a brace of poached pheasants on their front door, and driving around with a row of pheasant tail-feathers, stuck in potatoes, poking out of the back of his car.

Such stories serve to whet the appetite for game – even squirrel. Prue's presentation of the little vermin was simple but subtle. She tossed the jointed pieces in a smoking wok for a few minutes until nicely browned, and transferred them to a dish to finish in a warm oven.

She then deglazed her wok with a squeeze of lemon juice, a cup of game stock (which included a previous squirrel) and a dash of soy sauce. This sauce was finished with a little cream, and poured over the squirrel. The final, appropriate garnish was a sprinkling of chopped, toasted hazelnuts, 'which is,' as Prue put it, 'what made this squirrel grow up big and strong.'

I could see even before I ate it that this dish was going to be delicious. What surprised me was how tender and delicate the squirrel meat was as succulent as frog's legs, with a light, gamey flavour.

'Are we eating boys or girls?' I asked her.

'One of each,' she said. 'In fact it's a pity you didn't see the boy before I chopped him up. Their reproductive tackle is really quite impressive for such a small animal.'

A couple of older males – too tough, Prue reckoned, for the wok – had been subjected to her alternative preparation for squirrel; a fricassee. The long, slow cooking produced meat that melted in the mouth and a fine rich gravy. Here is Prue's definitive recipe:

Slow-braised squirrel with redcurrants and hazelnuts

Serves 4

2 squirrels, skinned, paunched and jointed; 600ml game or chicken stock; 1 onion stuck with 2 cloves; 1 carrot; 1 bay leaf; 1 glass red wine; 1–2 tsp redcurrant jelly; 50g redcurrants, blackberries, or morello cherries; 50g whole or halved hazelnuts, toasted; salt and pepper

Gently stew the squirrels in the stock with the onion, carrot, bay leaf and seasoning until tender (about 1 hour). Strain the cooking liquid, add the wine, and simmer to reduce, by up to three-quarters, to an intense sauce. Season with salt and pepper, and add a little redcurrant jelly to slightly sweeten the sauce. Remove the squirrel meat from the bones, and add back into the sauce. Add a scattering of the fruit, if available, and heat through.

Serve with rice, a simple salad, or lightly steamed greens, dressed with hazelnut oil and a scattering of hot toasted hazelnuts.

October 1993

Throughout my writing career I have tried to encourage people to take a more holistic view of the animals we use for meat. Other food writers and chefs, notably Jonathan Meades, Fergus Henderson and Matthew Fort, have done the same. Are we getting anywhere?

Well, offal is currently enjoying another wave of being fashionable on restaurant menus, and our 'Pig in a Day' course at River Cottage HQ, where we make everything from crispy roast tails to brawn with the head, is our most over-subscribed event. But until we see pig's trotters in major supermarkets and brawn on the deli counter, I'll have to conclude that there is still work to be done.

Here are some pieces where I stuck my neck out, as it were, in the hope of making new converts to the joys of offal . . .

Heads or tails?

Not everyone is happy to walk home with a pig's head in their shopping. I'm proud to be someone who is. I consider myself to be part of a movement to resist the final demise of offal from British cookery.

I don't just mean liver and kidneys. I'm talking about extremities and gory vitals – heads, ears, tails, trotters, brains, hearts, lungs, pancreas – the sort of things you would expect to turn up in Hannibal Lecter's larder.

These ingredients are cheap, nutritious and, in terms of the variety they offer in flavour and texture, tremendously exciting. Yet we barely cook with them any more, and most butchers have ceased to stock them. What went wrong?

Jeremy McClancy, a social anthropologist at Oxford University, blames the rise of the affluent society in the fifties and sixties: 'Basically, they were saying, "Look at us, we don't have to eat those nasty bits any more."'

This gastronomic posturing was facilitated by the boom in factory farming. Lean red meat became cheaper and cheaper, and soon practically everyone could afford not to eat offal.

It is ironic, then, that while we think we have given up offal, we may now be consuming more than ever, 'concealed' in pies and pâtés. It is this irony that fires those of us in the resistance to restore the reputation of offal in British cooking.

I say 'us' because, of course, I have some allies. Fergus Henderson, of St John Restaurant, just a bone's throw from Smithfield market, is a staunch promoter and talented preparer of offal in the British style. 'Our motto', he says, with rousing gesticulation, 'is nose-to-tail eating. We are celebrating all the joys of one beast. My favourite, I think, is brains, especially if you deep fry them. You've got this crunch outside, with a creamy cloud inside . . . mmm . . . they're just outstanding.'

Trendy restaurant-goers are one thing. But few of them – or any home cooks – are cooking much offal in their own kitchens. One reason for such reluctance may be the spectre of BSE. Well, with the ban on British cow's offal (except oxtail and tripe), I shall pass on calf's brains myself for the moment – although the Ministry of Agriculture maintains there is no threat of BSE from British meat. But there are always sheep's brains (better, if anything, than calf's) and a whole gallimaufry of porcine and ovine offal cuts to keep the inquisitive palate amused.

One problem is that butchers stopped stocking offal as demand for it died. The onus must be on the consumer to reverse this. When your butcher does stock much offal, buy it; when he doesn't, order it most will require no more than 24 hours' notice.

Once you have got your body part of choice, all you need are some good old-fashioned recipes – for dishes that don't disguise, but celebrate, the taste and texture of their spare-part ingredients. Here are a few . . .

Lamb's brains

Poach gently in water with 1 tbsp wine vinegar and a few stock vegetables for 20 minutes. Drain, cool, pat dry, dust with seasoned flour, and shallow fry in half olive oil, half butter, until golden brown. Throw in capers and fresh sage leaves for the last two minutes of frying. Serve on toast with pan juices.

Cheek

Stew very slowly in red wine, beef stock and stock vegetables, for 3–4 hours. Strain cooking liquor, add more wine, and reduce rapidly to a rich gravy. Cut the cheek into bite-size pieces and heat through in the gravy. Serve with very creamy mashed potatoes.

Fries (aka testicles, lamb's)

Blanch for 2 minutes in boiling water. Cool, then marinate in olive oil, red-wine vinegar and a sliced onion, for 3 hours, changing the marinade halfway through. Then slice, toss in well-seasoned flour and shallow fry in half butter, half olive oil, for 4 minutes each side. Serve with mustard and shallot vinaigrette.

Head (calf's or pig's)

Fromage de tête: have butcher split head in four. Clean head well and trim or burn off bristle. Simmer head slowly with one trotter and plenty of stock vegetables and herbs for at least 4 hours. Drain head, reserving stock. Remove all bones, roughly chop up meat and put in basin or loaf tin (with strips of blanched leek or carrot, if liked). Add 1 glass of cider or white wine to stock and reduce by half. Pour over meat to just cover, and leave to set. Serve with mustardy vinaigrette and Puy lentils.

Heart (sheep's or pig's)

Stuff bacon and prunes in cavity. Braise gently in strong beef stock with wine and onions for 2 hours, till tender. Reduce stock to make gravy at the end of cooking.

Sweetbreads (lamb's or calf's)

Soak in cold water for 3 hours. Then poach gently with stock vegetables for 20 minutes. Leave to cool. Pick over, removing membrane and gristle. Shallow fry as for brains above.

Tripe

Make a tomato sauce. Add cooked chickpeas and slices of spicy chorizo. Slice pre-blanched ox tripe and sautée gently for 6–7 minutes, then add to sauce and simmer for a few minutes. Serve with crusty bread.

March 1995

Headcase

I have a recurring dream. In it I flick off the top of my head to reveal my glistening pink brain which I then tuck into with a spoon. I eat the contents of my own skull as though it were a soft-boiled egg. This may sound rather disturbing but the dream isn't a nightmare. In fact it's one of the best meals I've had for ages.

A friend with an amateur interest in psychoanalysis tells me that the Freudian implications of this dream are very revealing. It's all to do with self-love, unnatural greed, and the fact that I make a living by using my brain to write about food.

Well, I'll pass on that for the moment but I don't mind admitting that brains – calf's brains and sheep's brains – are one of my favourite foods. They have a unique texture and flavour. Nothing else quite compares with that sweet, rich, creamy kernel of the young calf's head. I like them fried, nice and crispy on the outside, soft and creamy in the middle. I could eat them till the cows come home.

Unfortunately, although the mad cow scare has largely abated and been replaced with a more up-to-date paranoia over mad dogs, there is a residual resistance on the part of the public to feasting on calf's brains. Even the River Cafe, which once offered them almost daily on its menu, has practically stopped serving them.

The only place I know of in London where they still regularly crop up on the daily changing menu is the Blueprint Café, which is attached to the Design Museum near London Bridge. And very good they are too, deep-fried and served with a wonderfully piquant *salsa verde*.

These days, if I want brains, I usually cook them myself. Most good butchers will find calf's brains for you, if you give them a bit of notice. My favourite butcher in the whole world regularly has them in stock. Randall & Aubin, 16 Brewer Street, is one of those dusty old establishments that could only persist in Soho or the East End. Scrawny guinea fowl and white rabbits hang in the window, above trays of every kind of offal: liver, kidneys, trotters, trips, sweetbreads, lamb 'fries' (testicles) and, of course, brains.

The surly staff will almost certainly keep you waiting. If you get so much as a hello it probably means they've just won the pools. But once you get to talking meat, nothing is too much trouble. Last time I went there, I had to wait 15 minutes to get served, because the butcher was busy preparing a rack of lamb for a customer's dinner party. In it went black pepper, rosemary, and fresh garlic, which the butcher chopped by hand, before lovingly tying up the whole bundle with his fat, sausage-like fingers.

'Two sets of calf's brains, please,' I said, when he finally got round to me.

'Male or female?' he asked.

'What's the difference?'

'The male brain is bigger,' he replied, with the subtlest of glances at the lady behind me in the queue.

Brains are blissfully easy to prepare. First soak them in cold water in a basin, under a slowly running tap, for about half an hour. This removes excess blood.

Next, hold the brains under the tap, running your fingers through the crevices to remove the membrane and any remaining blood. Then simmer them gently in water, to which you have added a tablespoon of wine vinegar, for about 20 minutes.

Drain the brains and, when cool enough to handle, cut each of the lobes into two or three slices, roll in well-seasoned flour and then fry in a mixture of olive oil and butter, turning occasionally, until golden brown. Throw in a few fresh sage leaves, and/or capers, for the last couple of minutes of cooking.

Serve on toast, with a lemon wedge, and a simple green salad. Then you too can have dreams like mine.

October 1991

Brains have now become almost impossible to find. Indeed, for the best part of ten years, calf's and sheep's brains were effectively banned from sale in the UK, as a result of the BSE scare. But now, for sheep at least, the legislation has been relaxed – which means the recipe in the next article is theoretically achievable again.

Use your brains

How do you silence a curry bore? Ask him (it always is a 'him') if he's ever had a brain curry.

If the answer is yes, then, of course, you're in trouble. If the answer is no, then you can have the satisfaction of watching his jaw drop, while you say: 'Well, I have, and let me tell you, the way that soft creamy kernel of the young sheep's head combines with the pungency of fresh ginger and garlic . . .' At least, you can if you act on the information below.

Curry lovers who live in London should make an effort to get to one of the places where curry is cooked primarily for the discerning Indian palate. For easterners, Brick Lane is the best bet. For westerners, Southall has got the lot. (I particularly recommend Lahore at 162 The Broadway – bring your own beer.) You may find a brain (magaz) curry in a number of Indian restaurants. I urge you to try it. If you think you don't like brains, then I particularly urge you to try it.

Magaz curry

Serves 4

6 fresh lambs' brains; a few peppercorns; juice of half a lemon; 3 tbsp
corn oil; 1 medium onion; 100ml/4fl oz good meat stock; 400g/14oz
tin peeled plum tomatoes; 4 large cloves garlic, crushed; 2.5cm/1in
fresh root ginger, peeled and finely chopped; 1 small red chilli, finely
chopped; 2 tbsp garam masala (or better still, make the garam masala
by pounding in a pestle and mortar: half a cinnamon stick; 2 bay
leaves; 12 cardamom pods; 2 tsp cumin seeds; 1 tsp fenugreek;
2 cloves; a pinch of nutmeg); salt; freshly ground black pepper; chilli
powder; fresh coriander leaves, chopped; lime wedges

Clean the lambs' brains under a gently running tap, removing the
membrane and any blood clots. Poach the brains in simmering
water, with the peppercorns and lemon juice, for 25 minutes. Drain
and leave to cool.

Heat half the oil in a frying pan and add the onion. Sweat gently
until soft but not brown, then add the meat stock and tomatoes.
Turn up the heat and allow to bubble – stirring regularly so that it
doesn't catch on the pan – until well-reduced to a thick and pulpy
sauce. Set aside.

Roughly chop the brains. Heat the remaining oil in a clean pan,
and add the garlic. When it takes colour, add the ginger, chilli and
garam masala. Cook the spices for a few minutes, then add the
brains, and mix well. After a few minutes, add the tomato 'gravy'
(as the Indians call it). Season, mix well, simmer for about 5
minutes. Taste for seasoning (you can pep it up with extra chilli
powder if you like).

Sprinkle over the chopped coriander leaves just before serving.
Hand out lime wedges to squeeze over. Serve with plain boiled rice.

October 1993

I heard about the extraordinary fugu fish when I was a boy of nine, and was fascinated by the idea that anyone might risk death in pursuit of culinary ecstasy. Twenty years later, I put together a tidy package of Japan-based feature ideas in order to justify and pay for a trip there. But an adventure in pursuit of the taste of, and the truth about, this famous fish, was undoubtedly my main motive for going.

A fish to die for

In a busy restaurant in downtown Tokyo the sake is flowing. Two well-groomed businessmen face each other, kneeling, Japanese-style, across a low table. They are in a state of high excitement, talking shop, laughing and gabbling noisily. Suddenly one of them freezes, his face contorts, and his chopsticks clatter to the table. His companion gasps and a deathly hush descends as the other guests turn to stare. The staff freeze in horror.

After a couple of seconds, the contorted face relaxes into a broad grin. The diners break out into gleeful laughter, and the chef skulks back into the kitchen.

Why is this such a good joke? Because sometimes in Japan it is not a joke at all. For the restaurant is serving fugu, the puffer fish, a squat, ugly creature that can, when under attack, inflate itself like a football. Its second line of defence is its poison, 275 times deadlier than cyanide, which every year claims the lives of some dozen or so over-enthusiastic Japanese gourmets.

Despite the danger, fugu restaurants flourish in Japan's major cities, and the fish is regarded as the pinnacle of gastronomy – akin to Russia's caviar, France's foie gras, and Italy's white truffle. In price per serving, it outstrips the lot – a plate of fugu may go for $300 (about £206).

Any gourmet would reason that, to be worth the money, and the risk, fugu must be very good indeed. Ever in search of a new taste sensation, this particular gourmet has come to Tokyo, to find out if fugu is a fish worth dying for.

On my first evening, by way of a refresher course in handling raw fish with chopsticks, I seek out a sympathetic sushi bar in the neon bustle of the lively Roppongi district. I fall into conversation with the proprietor, who speaks good English and, though he doesn't serve it in his restaurant, happens to be something of a fugu fanatic. 'Do not worry,' he assures me, 'in a restaurant you should be safe. It is only when you eat the liver that you are in real danger, and it is prohibited to serve it by law.'

'I will tell you a story about a famous Japanese man who died from fugu. About 20 years ago,' he begins, with relish, 'Mitsugoro Bando, one of our most gifted kabuki actors, visited a fugu restaurant in Kyoto with a group of fellow actors. He wanted very much to eat fugu liver, and begged the chef to serve him. The chef agreed, but decided he must eat the liver with the actor and his guests.

'Those who ate just a single portion survived. But three of Bando's companions said they would not eat their liver, so the actor took their portions, too. Within an hour he was attacked by convulsions, and fell to the floor. His last words were: "I have eaten the death number." In Japan, you see, the number four is considered cursed.'

As I hear these words, I notice that four pieces of sushi are staring up from my plate. He sees them too, and laughs: 'Eat one quickly, and there will only be three.'

That night, as I lie awake, jet lag blending with culture shock in the mind's Magimix, I see images of clattering chopsticks and collapsing kabuki actors. The Emperor is not allowed to eat fugu. So why should I? With the contorted logic of these drowsy musings comes a mild thrill, creeping up from my toes. Even before a morsel of fugu has passed my lips, I have begun to partake of the strange cultural aura that surrounds the gastronomy of the deadly puffer.

The following evening, rehearsals over, my assignation with the fugu is for real. I meet Ken-ichi Hori, a benign Asiatic Bibendum in a green-brown suit, at the offices of Nikka Whisky, for whom he imports wine. He is a friend of a French friend, who has described him as a bon viveur, oenophile, gastronome and fugu aficionado. Most importantly, I have been assured that he is an all-round good egg *'qui aime un sake ou trois'*.

'So you are the brave Englishman,' he says, greeting me with a smile. He is taking me to a new fugu restaurant. 'It has only been open for ten days,' he tells me, 'and the chef is very young, but I hear he is one of the best in Tokyo.'

We take a taxi to the restaurant. I am introduced to the chef, Natsumetai, who, like Ken-ichi, is probably in his mid-thirties and, unlike Ken-ichi, is as thin as a rake. He invites us to sit at a wide bar, from which we can see him at work in his open kitchen. Ken-ichi explains the form: 'There is no menu,' he explains. 'The chef will prepare a number of courses, his specialities, and bring them to you as they are ready. He is just asking if there is anything you cannot eat.' 'Only fugu,' I am tempted to say.

The first course to arrive is tiny and beautiful – a little circle of marbled pink and orange, decorated with finely shredded white radish. 'This is a terrine of the fish's liver,' says Ken-ichi, almost causing me to drop my chopsticks. My mind races. The chef has no doubt been informed of my deep interest in fugu gastronomy, and how far I have travelled to sample his craft. He has prepared the liver illegally, especially for me. Am I about to be the first European victim of this dubious honour? 'Don't worry,' Ken-ichi assures me, 'it's not fugu. It's made from lumpfish liver, which is also considered a great delicacy.' It is Natsumetai's little culinary joke, to remind his customers of a lethal tradition, and provide a safe, legal alternative. The morsel, incidentally, is delectable.

The second course really is fugu – the shredded skin set in a jelly made from the fish's bones, flavoured with aromatic herbs and soy sauce. The jelly dissolves effortlessly in the mouth, leaving chewy strips of skin for the teeth to contend with – a novel and interesting oral experience.

Next comes the classic presentation of *fugu-sashi*. Tiny petals of raw fugu arranged like a chrysanthemum, cut so thin that the pale blue china is seen through the opalescent flesh. I take up two petals in my chopsticks, and dip them in a mixture of soy sauce, grated radish and *daidai* – a tiny relation of the orange.

In my mouth, the sauce has an appealing tang, but when this has gone I am left with raw fish of no instantly notable flavour. I chew the morsels. In spite of their fineness, they offer unusual resistance to the teeth. I move the meat around my mouth, in a thorough attempt to discern any subtle flavour. I cannot.

'What do you think?' asks Ken-ichi.

'Interesting,' I stall. 'Subtle.'

'Yes,' he agrees. 'It is not a strong taste.'

'Almost no taste at all?' I offer, a little more boldly now.

'In Japan,' Ken-ichi explains, 'some foods are prized very much for their blandness. Without taste, we can appreciate texture. Fugu is perhaps an extreme. The meat has almost no taste, but a very chewy texture.' The same could be said of rubber, I think, but it comes rather cheaper. Ken-ichi discerns the scepticism in my expression: 'I think perhaps it is difficult to understand if you are not Japanese.'

The ceremony of eating fugu is nothing if not holistic. Other parts of the fugu appear. Whole bodies of small fugu arrive deep-fried in the lightest of batters. The fleshy mouth, a delicacy known as 'the nightingale', is simmered with vegetables and mushrooms in a broth. The broth is then strained and served with rice balls.

After the broth I ask the chef if I may talk to his customers. He assents, and we are formally invited to join a table of four business-men. The chef brings us cups of *hirezake* – hot *sake* with a dried fugu fin floating in it, and Ken-ichi interprets as I ask them about fugu. All profess to partake of it regularly.

Predictably, perhaps, fugu is credited with aphrodisiac powers. One of my new companions explains the pulling power of the puffer in his charming but limited English: 'If one girl very beautiful, I want to invite to dinner, I am asking "Do you want to eat fugu?" I think she will go. And I think she will not refuse me.' With a grin he adds, 'After the dinner, I mean.'

'Do you feel the numbness of fugu?' his friend asks me. 'When we drink *hirezake* we can feel a tingling on the lips. It is caused by the tiny trace of poison that is found in the fin.' As he mentions it, I start to feel this sensation. I would like to dismiss it as psychosomatic, but it persists.

What about the taste of *fugu-sashi*, I ask them. Why is it so special? After a pause, I get an evasive answer, which takes up the fugu flavour mystery where Ken-ichi left off: 'To describe the deliciousness of *fugu-sashi* is almost impossible, because it is so subtle. It is like a search for taste which never ends.'

'Does the danger, and the price, add to or subtract from the pleasure of eating fugu?' I ask.

'We do not think it is very dangerous, but perhaps the knowledge that a fugu can kill a man adds to the excitement of eating the fugu. As for the price – well, that depends whether you like spending money. Most Japanese do!'

The fourth member of the party then speaks for the first time: 'Of course, today there is something missing from the menu,' he says. I know, of course, what he is talking about. I have heard, I tell him, that some restaurants still serve the liver, illegally. Have any of them tasted it? They look at one another, and shake their heads. 'We have wives and children,' says one, with a smile.

How could I find a chef who would serve me a liver, I ask, full of *sake* and bravado. They laugh. 'You will have to live in Japan a long time. Go to one fugu restaurant many times, over many years. Show the chef that you are a true gourmet, and understand everything about the fugu. Then perhaps, if the chef likes you, and trusts you, he may agree to serve you the liver. But unless you are Japanese, I do not think this will be possible.'

I am intrigued, and ask my informer how he knows about all this. 'I have a friend who eats fugu liver,' he replies.

'Perhaps I can meet him?'

Two days later, after a series of stressful and delicate telephone calls undertaken by an interpreter, I have arranged a rendezvous which I hope will finally explain the fugu's mysterious grip on the Japanese psyche. Over cappuccinos in a backstreet coffee shop, I meet a man who, once or twice a year, genuinely dices with death.

He is not the fat cat I am expecting, and sports no flash tailoring or glinting jewellery. But for a deep skin tone faintly suggestive of foreign travel, I would not pick him out from any clutch of Tokyo salarymen.

His greeting is polite but not friendly. He is the first person I have interviewed in Japan who has not presented a business card. 'The chef who prepares me fugu liver is a friend,' he says, by way of explanation for his caution. 'If he can be identified he may lose his licence.' He does not want to be photographed or named, and has made it clear to my interpreter that he cannot stay for long.

I pitch right in: 'What does the liver taste like?' 'Of course, I think it is very good,' he tells me, 'or I wouldn't eat it. But how do you explain a taste? It is rich, but delicate at the same time. Some compare it to the foie gras of France, but it is more subtle, more unusual.'

He feels unable to elaborate, so I ask him how it is prepared. 'In a paste, which is served with the *fugu-sashi* as an accompaniment. It really completes the dish. Without the liver, the fugu meat is very bland. You will know this if you have tasted it.'

I nod enthusiastically, in an attempt to communicate some modicum of gastronomic camaraderie, but he continues without acknowledging my gesture: 'The thing about fugu meat is that it has almost no fat at all. This is what gives it such a bland taste, and such an unusual dense texture. The liver, on the other hand, is extremely rich, containing almost all the fat reserves of the fugu. When the two come together, it is like a marriage – a very happy marriage.'

This simplicity is pleasing, an exalted and exotic version of the domestic bliss of our own Mr and Mrs Jack Sprat. But I know there is more to it than that. 'Are you frightened when you eat the fugu liver?' I ask.

'I trust the chef. He understands how to prepare the liver, and make it safe.'

But chefs have made mistakes, and people have died.

'You take your life in your hands when you cross the road,' he says, 'or when you fly in an aeroplane.' After a pause he adds, 'Personally, I don't think aeroplane food is worth dying for. I would prefer to die eating fugu.'

January 1994

My fugu quest was perhaps my most emotionally intense encounter with raw fish, but a more recent self-caught sushi feast definitely runs it close . . .

Seychelles, sharks and sushi

I learnt to dive 15 years ago, over almost six months of successive Thursday evenings, in a swimming pool in Swiss Cottage. My friend Jaimie learned to dive a few weeks ago, in just four days, on the island of Alphonse, in the Seychelles. While I was learning the vital skills of buddy breathing and buoyancy control back in 1989, the most diverting visual attractions on offer – my foretaste of great ocean adventures to come – were discarded corn plasters, matted balls of hair, and the grey–blue lines on the floor of the pool. In contrast, by the end of his second lesson in the Alphonse lagoon, Jaimie had a shoal of admiring parrot fish all to himself, and was on nodding terms with the local turtle.

My first open-water dive took place in a cold muddy quarry in Leicestershire, euphemistically called Stoney Cove, and the only fish I saw were a pair of gawping roach. Jaimie's first open-water dive was in the crystal waters of the stunning coral reef that surrounds the island, and within seconds of descending to the bottom, through small galaxies of shimmering reef fish, he found himself looking at a ten-foot nurse shark. I was with him at the time, and the experience of watching Jaimie watching the shark watching him actually made me laugh underwater. This was partly in sheer disbelief at the absurd contrast in our learning experiences, and the folly of my plodding progress all those years ago. But it was mainly because I knew that, despite the privilege of such an encounter on a first dive, the last thing Jaimie wanted to be looking at was a shark of any kind.

His fear of sharks is matched only by his fear of spiders (which, incidentally, is matched only by *my* fear of spiders). Although our dive guide, Norbert, had mentioned the possibility that we would see a shark, Jaimie had assumed he was joking. In fact, he told me afterwards that his first thought on seeing the shark, which was lying motionless in a sandy gully on the reef, was that it was a plastic one placed by the dive team as an elaborate practical joke. But when he noticed how the gills of the fish were rippling, and how its unmistakably sharky tail tilted occasionally to steady itself in the current, his fantasy rationalisation rapidly began to fade.

Despite my amusement, I felt obliged to do something to allay his fears. I had seen a few nurse sharks before, and I happened to know that, of all the sharks, they are the least likely to give divers any kind of grief. They are passive bottom feeders, who tend to lie up and sleep during the day, and swim lazily over the reef at night, munching the odd crab. They are the teddy bears of the shark world, in fact. In order to make this point, I swam towards the shark, with my hand stretched out towards its head, and made what I intended as gentle stroking motions a couple of feet away. At the same time, I looked over towards Jaimie and, with my non-stroking hand, made the thumb and finger circle that is the underwater signal for 'everything's okay'.

Jaimie's response was to invent an entirely new signal in the sub-aqua lexicon. It involved waving the extended index finger of his right hand vigorously from side to side, while shaking his head, and the meaning was clear: 'Listen, don't muck about. I can see that is a totally shark-shaped fish, so can we please swim rapidly in the opposite direction, now!'

Back on dry land, Jaimie reminded me that a principal objective of our week on Alphonse was that we should be eating the local fish, and not the other way round. In order to reassert our rightful place in the tropical food chain, we decided to take a day off from diving, and charter the island's serious fish-hunting boat, *Bijoutier*, in pursuit of a Seychellois fish supper. One of the finest eating fish in the Indian Ocean – and therefore probably the world – is the yellowtail tuna. In theory we were a couple of weeks too early to hook up with the seasonal run of yellowtail, but the odd fish had already been picked up before our arrival, so there was a faint hope of striking lucky. On the strength of that, I packed in my fishing box a tube of *wasabi*, a bottle of Kikkoman soy sauce, some pickled ginger, and a Tupperware box of vinegar rice. As an afterthought, I hacked down a large, banana leaf from the tree outside our bungalow, rolled it up, and stashed it in my rod case.

Jaimie took this level of preparation to be a cast-iron guarantee that the yellowtail, and indeed every other sushi-grade pelagic we might have hoped to encounter, would elude us for the entire day. And, for a while, it seemed like he might be right, but then 'Toooo-naah!' yelled Jude, our Seychellois fishing guide – jabbing his finger out to sea. A few hundred yards from the boat, there was a commotion in the water, all white splashes and sliver flashes. 'That's yellowtail,' said our skipper, Vaughan, calmly turning the boat towards the action.

I was having a private Attenborough moment at this fishy feeding frenzy, when I heard the pulse-quickening 'ZZZzzeeee!' of a reel gleefully pouring out line to a running fish. I grabbed the twitching rod and yanked on it. The fish yanked back, almost wresting the rod from my arms, and Jude helped me guide the rod butt into the 'stand-up' rig, a pivoting, swivelling rod holder designed to take some of the heat out of playing fast-running fish.

Mine wasn't quite the monster I'd first reckoned it, and after a few short surges it began, grudgingly, to come to the boat. Still, it was enough to make my arms ache. And it was a relief when Jude swung the steel-hooked gaffing pole over the side, and hauled on board a solid, quivering muscle of a fish. It was a yellowtail of about 30 pounds. 'A baby,' said Vaughan, mildly mocking my efforts. A few minutes later, it was Jaimie's turn to grunt, sweat and strain, and try to look nonchalantly tough. He made a showy job of it, I thought, but the full display was entirely justified when, after a struggle of a good 15 minutes, a second yellowtail, well over twice the size of mine, was hauled on board. 'How about lunch?' he asked, coolly. I was more than ready to oblige.

I laid out the banana leaf on the deck, and the over-optimistic eccentricity of my first-response sushi kit immediately came into its own. I only had my chunky diving knife to carve the fish with, but it was razor sharp, and did the job better than I expected. Individually moulded fingers of sushi rice seemed too formal, so I spread the rice in a thick layer over the banana leaf, and laid generous slices of tuna over it. I dabbed on little piles of *wasabi* and pickled ginger around the rice and between the fish. My sushi bar was open for business.

My God, it was good. The fish had an irresistible resistance, and a fullness to it, that I have never encountered in restaurant sushi – whose tuna, even when of the highest quality, has invariably been frozen. Alphonse is without doubt the ultimate Indian Ocean destination for diving and fishing, and for those who like to combine the two it is sheer heaven. What made it extra special was that, for a few brief moments at least, it also became the sushi capital of the world.

August 2004

The exotic and far-flung assignments are not always the most memorable. The next three pieces all stick in the mind, despite taking me no further than Reading!

Panel eaters

When I was young (by which I mean mid-single figures – still on the Nesquik and chocolate fingers) I knew what I wanted to be. It wasn't an unusual ambition. In fact, it was shared by the majority of my nursery school chums. We wanted to be taste-testers for Cadbury's. Or, according to variations in personal taste, for McVities, Lyons Maid, or Mr Kipling (an exceedingly good job, I believe).

Twenty years on, I have no idea whether any of my contemporaries from the class of 1970 made it in this field. But I recently met a lively bunch of lucky ladies who did.

This panel of taste-assessors are part-time employees of Reading Scientific Services Ltd (RSSL), formerly the research department of Cadbury Schweppes, now an independent consultancy for the food industry. This organisation is to be found in the Lord Zuckerman Research Centre, a breezeblock of a building attached to the campus of Reading University. RSSL is the place to go to if you want to discover the origin of the shards of glass in your baby food, or analyse a sample of Pot Noodle for traces of natural ingredients.

They also specialise in 'Quantitive Description Analysis' of food products, which is used 'to compare product prototypes with one another and with existing brands, and to assess the impact of recipe changes on sensory characteristics of a product'. In other words they answer the vital questions of the modern food industry: how do you make a Crunchie crunchier? or an Opal Fruit fruitier? or Shredded Wheat taste less like shredded junk mail?

This is where the lucky ladies come in. The tasting panel consists of ten Reading housewives (who better?) trained in the art of 'flavour note' detection.

For two mornings a week they subject anonymous samples of edible items to severe bouts of sniffing, licking, biting and chewing in a dedicated bid to investigate the full range of olfactory and oral sensations created by a product. Put simply, they eat for their daily bread.

I met them in a break between sessions. The research is confidential, so the brand names of the products they sample are kept from them (and me). But, in keeping with my childhood fantasy, I learnt that they had, that morning, been tasting chocolate bars. No surprise, then, to learn that they had enjoyed their morning's work. 'Today was fine,' said Annie, a bottled blonde who obviously enjoyed her chocolate. She admitted that the idea of being a taster had instantly appealed to a lover of food like herself. 'But some things aren't so much fun to taste. Fizzy drinks, for example.' The rest of the panel murmured agreement: 'They make you feel so full . . . sort of bloated . . . and give you wind . . .'

After joining the ladies in a palate-cleansing snack of water and dry biscuits (hardly a perk of the job) I was able to participate in a mock tasting session. This was not for real and no secrecy was required, so the ladies had been asked what they wanted to taste. Their choice confirmed my suspicion that they were all sweet-tooths at heart: they plumped for ice-cream bars.

The session that followed was the first stage of the testing of any new product or group of similar products – Descriptive Vocabulary Derivation. Initial tasting of the samples was followed by a brainstorming (or was it palate-storming?) session, the aim of which was to provide a full vocabulary to describe all aspects of the product in four categories: Odour, Flavour, Texture and Aftertaste.

I could tell they'd played this game before. And no doubt they could tell I hadn't. On Odour, for the Bonanza bar, I came up with nothing less obvious than 'roasted peanuts' and 'caramel'. Meanwhile the regular panel had no trouble at all in discerning such blatant smells as 'fruity, nearly pineapple' and 'bonfire' as well as the elusive, if not meaningless, 'sweet'. 'I got cardboard,' announced Elizabeth, when it came to Taste. 'Definitely,' agreed Jane. Aftertaste provided such gems as 'mouthcoat' (self-explanatory) and 'tooth-etch' (that unmistakable feeling you get when some corrosive foodstuff has seared the enamel off your incisors). My own minor triumph came when I described the aftertaste of a Figaro as 'fatty'. At least two of the panel agreed with me.

Clearly these ladies had a whole mouthful of taste-buds, and the terminology to match. Someone ought to send them out to do their stuff in the country's top restaurants. Not *Punch* though. Or I might be a couple of canapés short of a free lunch.

August 1990

Not bloody likely lads

Last Sunday morning I had the great honour of being a judge in a competition to find the best Bloody Mary in London. The venue was Joe's Brasserie, in the Wandsworth Bridge Road; the sponsors, Absolut Vodka (which every barman knows is the best). Some clever chap with red glasses and a spotty bow-tie – he might almost be me – had therefore decided the event should be called 'Abso-bloody-lutely'.

The chef at Joe's had prepared a fine pre-competition brunch of strong coffee, fresh croissants, kedgeree, sausages, bacon, scrambled eggs and mushrooms – the works. This was just as well, as being true professionals, my co-judge (the *Evening Standard*'s stalwart restaurant critic Fay Maschler) and I had both gone out and got completely legless the night before – separately, I should add, and her no doubt in a more respectable and lady-like manner than myself. But truly hungover we both were, and therefore perfectly qualified to pro-nounce judgement on the pickmeupability of these barmen's (there were no barwomen) versions of the famous cocktails.

As the bartenders (they like to be called that) gathered, the banter began, and it was clear they were in boisterous and competitive spirit: 'Don't forget the vodka like you normally do at your place!' . . . 'Now this is a fresh lemon, you probably haven't seen one of those before.' Many had brought with them secret ingre-dients. Those who had come unarmed could choose from a wide range of condiments, including fresh horseradish, chilli, sherry, several types of mustard, paprika, limes, plus the more usual Worcestershire sauce, Tabasco and celery salt.

My worry was that, in a tasting of ten Bloody Marys, after the first two or three my taste-buds would be blitzed by the spices and rendered incapable of discerning further subtleties. And indeed, the first one was so blindingly hot (it turned out it was made with chilli vodka) that I feared I might have to retire hurt. But after a mouthful of kedgeree and a couple of cigarettes to cleanse the palate, I was ready for the next nine. In the event, all ten were so completely different that I need not have worried.

Most striking of the 'clever' ingredients adulterating the mix were such curiosities as fresh carrot juice, fresh orange juice, beef con-sommé, crushed cucumber, grated onion and dried chillies. These were all highly discernible, but in most cases served only to emphasise the difference between this novelty and the classic Bloody Marys we were actually looking for. Eccentric decorations included chopped chives and, winning a prize for the most ostentatious display of bartender bad taste, a garnish of an olive, a hard-boiled quail's egg, a cherry tomato, all kebabed on a wooden skewer, and topped with a plume of dill weed.

I'm happy to say that the judges were unanimous in their verdict. Amid loud cries of 'It's a fix', the home team bartender, Giles Boden, was pronounced the winner by a clear seven points. It wasn't a fix, honest. The simple truth is that Mr Boden's remarkably uncontroversial recipe happens to make a bloody good Bloody Mary. And here it is:

The Joe's Brasserie Bloody Mary, by Giles Boden

$1\frac{1}{2}$ tbsp dry sherry; 190ml vodka; 2 tbsp fresh lemon juice; 2 tsp Worcestershire sauce; $\frac{1}{3}$ tsp creamed horseradish; 6 drops Tabasco; 4 cubes ice; squeeze of lime; freshly ground black pepper; good shake celery salt.

Stir the above ingredients in a glass. Top up with tomato juice. Add the ice, lime, 4 twists of pepper and celery salt, and garnish with a stick of celery and a straw.

Finally, the wearing of an outlandish pink ruffled evening shirt while serving your customers also helps a lot.

November 1991

The rations are coming

According to our man in the Gulf, Gerard Evans, journalists over there are having a tough time tracking down a decent meal and an even tougher one finding something agreeable to wash it down with. My sympathy for them is a bit limited. Their plight is as nothing compared with the real heroes. For Our Boys, the Gulf campaign is unlikely to be much of a gastronomic adventure. At best, they may be able to lay their hands on a decent *kabsa* (spicy lamb stew) during one of their rare periods of leave in Bahrain. Otherwise, they will be at the mercy of the force's catering corps.

But things really get bad for Our Boys when they go out on patrol, or advance on the enemy to engage in battle. I'm not just talking about the obvious dangers of bullets and bombs. It's a pretty rough time for the discerning squaddie's palate too. For once they leave behind the security of their base camps (where, to be fair, the catering corps are said to do a better job than most countries, including France) all they have to sustain them – and amuse their tastebuds – is one emergency ration pack every 24 hours. For amateur army aristologists, it's not a lot to go on.

The contents of a standard army ration pack, which is the same for all three services, has not changed much over the years. 'Breakfast' is a tinned bacon roll or beefburger, porridge oats and a chocolate drink. 'Main Meal' is all tinned. The contents may vary, but you are likely to get a tinned meat dish such as a stew (with vegetables) or, particularly popular, a steak and kidney pudding. For afters, you'll get a tinned fruit cocktail – or peaches – in syrup. Most coveted in the ration pack is the snack bag, the contents of which are listed in the pack 'menu': 'Ham spread; Biscuits – brown; Biscuits – fruit-filled; Chocolate – full cream; Chocolate-covered caramels; Nuts and raisins; Dextrose tablets – lemon.' The emphasis, you may have noticed, is on energy-giving high sugar foods. The notoriously sweet-toothed squaddies love them.

To my great surprise, so did I. The 'Biscuits – brown' are particularly palatable. Dry and very crunchy, they are slightly sweet, and taste like a cross between Rich Tea biscuits and Winalot. You get two packets of six, so they amount to a fairly significant hunger postponer.

The American ration packs are considered most inferior. They are smaller, and give only about half the calorific value. The one I tried had a most unpleasant main dish of 'Turkey – diced with gravy'. This gelatinous sludge came out of a slime-green vacuum pack, and was no better hot than cold. You get no chocolate either. No wonder that out in the Gulf these packs exchange for British ones at the rate of up to ten for one.

It would be quite wrong to assume that that the ration packs are beneath gastronomic assessment, or that the soldiers don't care what they eat. According to an MoD source, many of the lads take their own condiments into battle to improve the R&R function of their hastily snatched mealtimes. Worcestershire sauce and Tabasco are highly sought after, and a squaddie with a bottle of either is likely to make plenty of friends or, if he is the entrepreneurial type, extra chocolate, sugar or fags.

Soldiers in search of a little culinary variety do not stop there. Using only the contents of the mess tin, a number of novel recipes have been devised. One of these is even acknowledged in the menu/cooking instructions that come with every pack. In preparing your breakfast porridge oats, it is suggested 'You can also add chocolate drink mix and/or nuts and raisins to make a variety of breakfast meals' and 'you can save a portion of your rice to serve with your apple dessert'. But undoubtedly the most commonly prepared recipe, a child of necessity, is a rather less genteel affair. When the action hots up, and hunger is raging alongside battle, vital fuel must be consumed as quickly as possible. In this situation, the traditional solution is to empty the entire contents of the ration pack (minus, perhaps, matches and loo paper) into a mess tin, and stir. If time allows, it can be heated up. 'It's surprisingly good,' said my source at the MoD, 'sort of sweet and sour'.

By way of a contribution to this spirit of culinary adventure in the face of enemy fire, I have been experimenting with the ration-pack contents, and endeavouring to come up with an original, exciting, and, above all, tasty recipe. After slaving over a hot mess tin for many hours, I think I've cracked it. May I present, as a tribute to chocolate-loving, sweet-toothed soldiers of all ranks, my very own Gulf gâteau. *Bombe appetit*, as they say in Iraq.

Gulf gâteau

1 pint boiling water; 2 sachets instant coffee; 5 brown biscuits; 2 sachets beverage whitener; 2 packets Rolos; ½ a bar of chocolate; 1 packet fruit and nuts.

Make an extra strong cup of black coffee with most of the boiling water and the instant coffee. Soak 4 of the biscuits in the coffee until soggy. This is best done in a mess tin – or helmet.

Mix the rest of the water with the whitener in a small mess tin. Add the Rolos and chocolate and heat gently, stirring to melt. When melted, add the nuts and raisins and stir in.

Lay 2 of the soggy biscuits in the bottom of a small mess tin. Pour half the chocolate mixture over the top. Make another layer with 2 more coffee-soaked biscuits, and cover with the remaining chocolate. The fifth biscuit, unsoaked, should be crushed to crumbs (use your bayonet), and sprinkled over the top.

Serve whilst warm, or keep till later (when it will probably still be warm).

February 1991

The following article put me on record as being pro-legalisation (of cannabis), during the Independent on Sunday's *campaign to bring this about. Its limited success was, perhaps, to contribute to the reclassification of cannabis as a class C drug, but it did not achieve the arguably more worthwhile goal of lifting the restrictions on research into the medical use of cannabinoids.*

After it was published, I received a charming 'thank you' letter from an elderly gentleman who had begun to use home-made hash brownies as a pain-relieving treatment for his wife's severe arthritis. He said she was unquestionably feeling the benefit and felt sure that medically controlled cannabis treatments had the potential to relieve a huge amount of suffering and lamented the government's continued inaction over the matter.

Making a hash of it

Frank Dobson, Health Secretary, and other Cabinet ministers have criticised the *Independent on Sunday*'s cannabis campaign on the grounds that we are encouraging smoking. But cannabis can be a harmless addition to food – as with these hash brownies, for example.

Hash brownies can be potent, and should be eaten in moderation (initially no more than one to two per person), and not offered to unwitting innocents. The flavour imparted by hash to biscuits, cakes and other recipes is a strong one, and it is not to everyone's taste. The inclusion of coffee, rum and quality dark chocolate in this recipe prevents the flavour of hash becoming too overpowering. The very black sticky, resinous types of hash have a particularly harsh flavour, and can also cause mild stomach upsets. They'll do the job, but more crumbly varieties, such as Red Leb, are preferable.

Hash brownies

Makes approximately 12 brownies

115g/4oz unsalted butter; 2–4g/⅛–1/16oz hash (depending on the quality of the product, and the desired effect); 200g/7oz good dark chocolate (such as Green and Black's organic); 1 tbsp strong, black coffee; 1 tbsp rum; 115g/4oz caster sugar; 2 eggs; 55g/2oz ground almonds; 55g/2oz self-raising flour; 55g/2oz walnut pieces (optional); 55g/2oz seedless raisins (optional)

Pre-heat the oven to 160°C/Gas mark 3. Grease, flour and line a 20cm x 25cm/8in x 10in rectangular cake tin, or similar.

Put the butter in a medium-sized heavy-bottomed saucepan, and place over a low heat. As the butter starts to melt, crumble the hash into it as finely as possible (using a lighter to soften it if necessary).

Then add the chocolate, in small pieces, coffee and rum, and stir gently over a low heat until the chocolate is melted and the mixture thoroughly blended. Beat in the sugar, then the eggs, then the ground almonds, and then fold in the flour. Stir in the walnuts and/ or raisins, if used. Spread the mixture into the lined tin, and bake in the pre-heated oven for 35–40 minutes. They should have a light crust on top, but still be a bit gooey in the middle.

They are delicious, and speedily effective, when eaten warm, but can be kept for up to a week in the fridge.

October 1997

The substance with which we food writers self-medicate is wine, and sometimes the very anticipation of it can befuddle the senses, even before a drop is imbibed.

No head for figures

When I was about 14, I did one of those so-called vocational aptitude tests that, in conjunction with an interview with a scary stranger, is supposed to help you work out what you want to do with your life.

The chief findings of this rather stressful ordeal were that I was in the bottom five per cent of the country at mental arithmetic, and wanted to work with animals. It was hinted that a career as a vet might be beyond me, presumably because of the risk that I might give St Bernard-sized doses of doggy medication to hapless chihuahuas. The conclusion of the independent assessor was that maybe I could work in a pet shop, provided I wasn't allowed to operate the till.

At college, I played darts, and my inability to subtract any two-figure number without a nought or a five at the end from any three-figure number without the same became legendary. However, I did play a lot of darts, and eventually I improved.

But it wasn't until a few weeks ago that the mathematical chip on my shoulder was finally expunged. I appeared on *Celebrity Countdown* on Channel 4 where my opponent was a fellow foodie, the very lovely Jilly Goolden. We were even-stevens on the wordy bit, but when it came to the maths I astonished myself by getting both teasers bang on the target number. I think Jilly was a more gracious loser than I was a winner. I fear I looked terribly smug. Frankly, I was back in the classroom, and it was all I could do to restrain myself from turning to Jilly and slapping the side of my face while taunting 'Der-brain, der-brain!'

Last week I was recounting the story of my great victory to my girlfriend, Marie, as we drank kirs at the bar of the Paris restaurant, Laperouse. 'This show started in France,' she told me (she is French). '*Les Chiffres et les lettres* – it's been going for years.'

'Nonsense,' I countered, 'it's another English format, bought by the French, just like *N'Oublie pas ta brosse à dents*.'

'Boll-ox,' she said, with delightful, equal emphasis on both syllables.

I decided to drop the matter, before it became vicious, and started to look at the wine list. (It turns out she is quite right.)

It was a special occasion for us, and Laperouse is a very special restaurant – perhaps the most romantic in Paris, which is saying something (the Train Bleu at the Gare de Lyon would be another contender). I'm not going to describe the place for you, because that would spoil the surprise. I'll just say that it's old, and that Balzac and Proust went there a lot. Go there with someone you love, and be amazed.

So I was looking at the wine list, after something just a bit lush. Marie had ordered *jarret de veau à l'ancienne* and I was expecting *coq au vin Laperouse*, so a hefty Bordeaux seemed in order. My eye came to rest on a Château Petrus 1983, on offer for an astonishingly reasonable Fr5,500 (a little over £65, I calculated, at the current exchange rate). I ordered it from the waitress, who nodded and smiled with, I felt, deep approval, and went and whispered to the sommelier. She returned to us immediately, and offered us another kir on the house. As she was pouring it, the sommelier appeared and showed us, with some pride, the Petrus, its ageing label emblazoned with the famous gothic script. 'Classy place,' I thought to myself, 'where else but Paris?'

But Marie sensed something was going on. 'Have you ordered something expensive?' she asked.

'Well, a bit extravagant,' I confessed, 'but it'll be worth it. I promise.'

'How much?' she asked.

'Don't worry about it.'

'How much?' she demanded.

'If you really need to know, about £60.'

'Are you sure?' she persisted, 'there were an awful lot of noughts on that part of the wine list.'

An uneasy feeling started to creep up from my toes. I reached over for another look at the wine list. Fr5,500. Divide by eight point five. That's, er, not £65. More like £650. I blushed as I raised a hand sheepishly to attract the waitress's attention. 'Er,' I asked her, 'has the sommelier opened the bottle yet?'

'I'm not sure,' she said, looking me in the eye, 'I'll go and see.'

She seemed to walk ever so slowly across the room and through the door the sommelier had recently exited. I strained for the sound of a cork popping. She returned with a slightly arched eyebrow – to keep me guessing. 'He has not opened it yet,' she said, challengingly. 'Would you like to change your mind?'

'Yes,' I said. 'I'm afraid I would,' and in a misguided attempt not to lose too much face, I reordered a lesser bottle from the same year, for a respectable Fr810. Still the most expensive wine I have ordered in a restaurant. And, I'm sorry to say, a bit of a disappointment.

The food, however, was sumptuous, in the classic French mould. We both started with *quenelles de la mer parfumées aux truffes*, and each plate carried a worryingly large but, it turned out, feather-light pair of poached mousses, based on simple white fish but with a sweetness that I would guess came from the inclusion of scallops. They came with a rich cream-based sauce extravagantly garnished with slivers of black truffle, and we both loved them.

Our main courses were both unfinishably huge. My *coq au vin* was cooked for so long, and with so much heavily reduced red wine, that it was as black as oxtail stew and almost as rich. A few mouthfuls were all I could manage. I preferred Marie's veal, meltingly tender, with a lighter, herb-scented *jus*.

The smart thing to do would have been to share a main course, because the puddings were also huge. Marie had *pain perdu et ses petits pots de crème* – a brioche soaked in *crème anglaise* and flashed under the grill, served with little pots of vanilla, chocolate and hazelnut custard. She liked it a lot, but was soon distracted by my *soufflé Laperouse*, flavoured with Grand Marnier, which achieved the perfection of being crusty on the outside, light and moussey under the crust, and completely gooey and saucy in the middle.

By now we had both forgotten about maths and money, and agreed, with an extravagant confidence borrowed from our surroundings, that this was undoubtedly the best soufflé in the world. I didn't dare look at the bill, but however much it was, it was worth it.

June 1998

My Lapland experience, described below, was genuinely an inspiration – both as an adventure in new tastes, and, more profoundly, as an example of a culture that has lost neither the art of living in tune with its landscape, nor the respectful, holistic good sense of using every last part of its primary livestock provider – the reindeer.

A reindeer is not just for Christmas

The day I taste my first reindeer could hardly be further from Christmas. It's late June, within a week of the longest day of the year. I'm in Lapland, where the days are not just long, but technically endless. The sun doesn't set. It just bounces along the horizon in a teasing kind of way, as if to say, 'You must be shattered . . . fancy a kip?' Then, just when you're nodding off, it soars upwards again with an 'oh, no you don't . . .'

We are on a large floating wooden raft, edged with wooden rails, with its own bolted-down wooden tables and benches, a wooden roof and even a little wooden sauna hut. On the middle of the wooden floor is a huge, free-standing cast-iron, pot-bellied barbecue, stoked with blazing logs. Were it not for the ready supply of water all around us, the designer of this craft would seem like a serious contender for a Darwin Award. But the Lapps, I am to discover, know wood and fire intimately, and handle both with innate understanding and great skill.

The river down which we are gently chugging is clear and fairly shallow, about 200 metres wide, edged with reedy dunes, leading back to pine-forested gentle slopes. On cue, as the skewers of marinated meat are laid on a grill above the fire, a pair of shabby reindeer (they moult in June) amble from the edge of the pines 100 metres ahead of us. They make their way down to the river, walk into the water up to their shoulders, swim across the deeper channel in the middle, their antlers waggling above the ripples, and calmly walk out again on the other side.

We've touched down at Kittila airport scarcely an hour before. We've seen real live reindeer, and now I'm about to eat a real dead one. I bite on the cube of lightly charred meat and chew. It's soft and tender, and less dry than most other deer species, even after the fierce heat of the barbecue. It tastes pleasantly of juniper – the principal flavouring of much of Lappish cooking, both meat and fish.

I'm sitting beside my hostess, a delightful Lappish lady called Paivikki Palosaari, who runs the lodge where I am staying, and does most of the cooking too. I can see she wants a pretty quick verdict, so before I have a chance to swallow, I'm nodding enthusiastically and making appreciative noises, 'mmm . . . mmm . . . derriffous'.

The meat's unique qualities, Paivikki tells me, are a product of the reindeer's diet and lifestyle. A supremely adapted selective grazer, it eats over 100 different types of wild plant according to the season. It's also a meticulous conserver of energy, rarely breaking into a run except in flight from predators. So the slow-growing muscle has a chance to develop the subtle grains of fat – the 'marbling' so prized in the best beef – that most of its cervine relatives are lacking.

She goes on to explain what a resource the reindeer is for the Lapps; how they eat everything but the skin and antlers, which of course have other uses. It's smoked, stewed, salted and made into pâté. Reindeer sausages are a perennial favourite and reindeer salami is stuffed in a natural casing made from its own intestines. Its liver is as rich and mild as calf's. Its tongue slow-cooks to a melting tenderness. Its blood makes a kind of black pudding called 'blood bread' and its milk is so thick, creamy and sweet it's eaten on its own for tea.

As we're chatting and eating, a long canoe approaches our raft, with a sumptuously bearded fellow at the back, steering with a little outboard motor. As he pulls alongside, I see he is wearing felt and reindeer from head to toe. His reindeer-skin boots look particularly cosy. The canoe turns out to be a traditional Lappish dug-out, generously lined with loose reindeer skins.

He's called Tapsa, and looks like Father Christmas on his summer holidays, which, it turns out, is not so far off the mark. He is a sort of 'professional Lapp', and an associate of Paivikki, whose job it is to ensure that her guests have as authentic a Lappish experience as possible. But he's not faking it. In the winter he drives sleigh safaris with both reindeer and huskies, in the spring and summer he traps fish on the river, and in the autumn he gathers wild mushrooms for Paivikki's kitchen.

Tapsa lashes his canoe alongside the raft, and we zig-zag across the river, stopping at rocks and weedbeds where he has laid his fish traps. In all of them are dozens of wriggling, tiger-striped, hump-backed perch, a few grayling, with their sail-shaped fins, and the odd small but muscular croc-jawed pike. All are killed, regardless of size, because they all are to be eaten.

It's nearly midnight as the raft heads back upstream to the jetty, though the sun suggests late afternoon. Paivikki and Father Christmas set about gutting and scraping the catch, dipping them occasionally in a bucket of river water. When the bucket is emptied into the river, a swirl of shimmering scales dance in the wake of the outboard.

The next day I spend the morning fly-fishing on the river. I catch a few half-kilo grayling, which I kill and keep as I know they'll be put to good use. But the wild Lappish salmon eludes me. Luckily my incompetence has been anticipated, and when I break for lunch and return to the *rantamokki* (a log-built fishing lodge overlooking the river) I find my fishing host, Kopi, another friend of Paivikki, brandishing a beautiful salmon he caught the day before.

Inside the *rantamokki* are various fireplaces configured in different ways. On and around them are all sorts of spits, racks, trivets, pans, kettles, cauldrons and hot plates, all fashioned out of black cast iron. The Lapps are truly the masters of every variation of wood-fired cookery, and the way in which my host deals with the salmon is a case in point.

He cuts a long, fat fillet from the fish and lays it skin-down on a fresh plank of wood – birch, he tells me. He pushes the blade of his hunting knife through the flesh, and gives it a couple of taps with a stone to make a notch in the plank. Then he cuts a few short splints from the edge of another scrap of wood. He pushes these through the slits in the fish, so their sharp points find the notches he made with his knife, securing the fillet to the plank. It's taken over to the central fire, and simply leaned on a trivet, at an angle of about 60 degrees.

Within a minute the surface of the salmon flesh is taking colour, and the fatty juices are starting to run. The fish is seasoned with salt and a few twists of a mill containing peppercorns and allspice berries. In 15 minutes, it's a tawny golden colour, just cooked through. My appetite is at the point of twitching anticipation. I taste the fish – half smoked, half grilled, beautifully seasoned – and it is the best salmon I have ever eaten.

Over the next couple of days, the feasting is interrupted only by the odd fishing trip, sauna, and swim in the river. The last night is billed as a special farewell dinner. Paivikki promises to pull out all the stops. But it's hard to see how she can top what we've had so far.

She explains the plan. We are going to spit-roast a whole haunch of reindeer in the fire that has been blazing outside the lodge almost non-stop since we arrived. Paivikki takes the huge haunch and lays it on a double sheet of greaseproof paper. On and around it go thick slices of streaky bacon, root vegetables, and great sprigs of juniper and bay leaf. I help her wrap the parcel in layer after layer of wet newspaper, it's all bound up with thick garden wire, and we carry it outside. The burning logs are scraped to one side of the fire, and Tapsa digs a metre-wide hole right underneath where the fire was blazing. The parcel goes in, the smouldering logs are raked back over it, and the fire is rekindled with fresh wood.

I have been invited to prepare a course, and I have asked Paivikki to find me some reindeers' tongues. I'm simmering them gently in a liquor of water, wine, vegetables, and juniper, which will be reduced to make an intense sauce. Paivikki asks me how long I'm going to cook them and I tell her about three hours. She shakes her head and tuts, 'These are much more delicate than cows' tongues. They'll be done in an hour and a half.' I'm sceptical as I imagine the tongues at work on those hundreds of rough and thorny Lappish plants. They must be tough old muscles. But I keep a eye on them as they simmer gently in their stock, and she's quite right. In just 90 minutes they pass Mrs Beeton's classic test for boiled tongue: 'so tender that a straw would penetrate it'.

The first night's catch of perch, grayling and pike turn up as an aperitif, variously salted, cured and smoked, and served with endless glasses of ice-cold Lappish vodka. The next course is also fish – a soup of salmon with cream and great handfuls of dill. Rich, aromatic and wonderful. Then comes my dish of tongues, skinned, sliced, and glazed with the rich, winey reduction. Better – tenderer, tastier – than calves' tongues, I think. A couple of tongue sceptics at the table claim to have been converted, which feels good.

Three courses in, and we're all pretty daunted at the prospect of the spit-roast reindeer haunch, but we gather round as Paivikki starts to unwrap the charred paper parcel. She gets to the meat, and it looks and smells delicious. But she doesn't look happy. She prods it a couple of times, and says it isn't ready yet. It needs to go back in the fire, for at least a couple more hours.

She's distraught and I think she may burst into tears. We all reassure her that it's just as well, that we've already had a wonderful dinner, and would struggle to manage the haunch anyway. It's true because we really are completely stuffed. Eventually she starts to accept our solace, then says, with a weak smile, 'You're not too full for my little pudding, I hope.' We all laugh, and reassure her . . . no, not too full for that . . .

It's roast cheese – a very fresh cow's curd, slightly sweetened, pressed in a mould, and then baked in a wood-fired oven until speckled brown – served with a compote of wild cloudberries. The sheer deliciousness of the concoction helps me find space for a second helping.

The next morning the untouched haunch of venison is on the breakfast table, now cooked to Paivikki's satisfaction, but cold. She carves me a slice, and serves it up with a spoon of the bittersweet cloudberry compote.

I have been utterly seduced by her stunning Lappish hospitality. In just a few days, I have been inducted into a culinary culture that is more holistic, more robust, more in touch with its wild and natural heritage, more resourceful, generous, honest and deeply touching than any I have visited before. So I guess by now I am a little biased. But I really do think this breakfast haunch of reindeer is the best cold meat I have ever tasted. And I ask for another slice.

December 2002

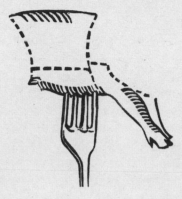

Meat and Right

I have a dream that, one day,
a man shall be judged by
the contents of his
shopping basket

As far as the ethics of food goes, animal welfare is obviously right at the heart of the matter. And if we're going to make a difference, it's clear there'll have to be a fight. As I see it, trying to change the disgusting way we produce chickens, for fast food and the supermarkets, is currently the front line.

Death of a chicken

I wrung a chicken's neck this morning. A cockerel's neck, to be precise. I've probably done a couple of dozen or so, in the last few years, since I regularly started raising my male chicks for the pot. And I'm getting better at it.

The technique, which I gleaned from various old poultry-rearing manuals, requires grasping the legs of the bird firmly in one fist (my right) and the head firmly between the middle fingers of the other hand (my left), and then pulling the two hands apart, firm and fast, in the opposite direction from each other (legs up, head down seems to work well). It has to be done with confidence and determination, as the neck vertebrae actually need to part company for the dispatch to be efficient. Provided this is achieved, the effect is fairly instant, and the bird is immediately rendered quite lifeless, bar the odd twitch.

That may all sound a bit grisly to some. But I feel pretty good about raising and killing my own meat birds. Relatively speaking, that is. I think I've got their death down to a minimum of stress and suffering – in other words, it compares favourably, in terms of speed and pain, to the death of most birds at the hands (or teeth, or claws), of a creature that intends to eat them. And of course that's how almost every bird, wild or domesticated, meets its end.

But with my cockerels what I feel best about is not so much the way they die, as the way they live. They scamper about in a grassy field, strutting their stuff and pecking the living daylights out of the grass, bugs and slugs, along with the corn and maize mix we scatter for them. In other words, they spend all day doing properly chickeny stuff. And as a result, they taste properly chickeny at the end of it all.

Compare and contrast the standard broiler chicken, reared in the millions of millions around the world (including around 800 million a year here in the UK alone). It lives a short, uncomfortable and wholly unnatural life. The resulting bland, tasteless pith, like papier mâché without enough glue, is a malleable food commodity that is, with the addition of the full battery of artificial flavourings, conveniently moulded and extruded into all kinds of ready-made meals and fast-food products. And it accounts for an astonishing 98 per cent of all the chicken meat we eat in this country.

For those of you who haven't heard the worst about intensive chicken farming, let me summarise briefly: a unique breed of chicken called the Ross Cobb, genetically engineered over hundreds of generations to be inherently obese, is raised from an egg to a two-kilo bird in a mere six weeks (it would take one of my cockerels getting on for 20 weeks to make that weight). At the end of this process, each bird has a space on the floor slightly smaller than an A4 sheet of paper.

The litter of woodshavings in the shed is not changed once during the six weeks. The resulting dung is so high in ammonia that, from four weeks on in the cycle, many of the birds suffer serious abrasions, known as 'hock burns' on their legs.

Every day in the sheds, dozens of dead birds, usually expired from stress-induced heart attacks, are removed from the sheds. Premature mortality is measured in 'acceptable percentages' of five to ten per cent per crop. Across the industry, that's well over 50 million chickens that die before they reach their slaughter weight. (In theory, these birds are banned from the human food chain and go to make pet food, fertiliser, or maggots for anglers. But it is far from rare for this meat to be illegally recycled for human consumption.)

Compassion in World Farming have argued that the broiler bird is such a genetic freak that it is impossible to raise it on this regime without inevitable suffering in a significant (over 30 per cent) proportion of the population. To farm it at all, they maintain, should technically be illegal under EC animal welfare legislation.

They point to the undisputed fact that the parent birds in the Cobb breeding programme (the ones that lay the eggs that hatch into the broiler birds) are reared on a completely different feed regime – effectively a starvation diet, that leaves them in a permanent state of hunger. This is because, on the same diet as their children are destined to receive, they would invariably die of obesity before they could ever reach sexual maturity.

You may or may not have heard all this before. If you have, then why are you (98 per cent of you) still buying this rubbish? You didn't know you were? Be in no doubt, that unless someone is specifically, loudly, unambiguously taking the trouble to tell you otherwise (by using the words 'free-range' or 'organic' on a label or menu), ALL the chicken you eat is made in this way.

What's bizarre is that we seem to have a completely different set of moral scruples about laying hens than we do about meat birds. The battle on behalf of the poor beleaguered laying hen has, over the last 30 years or so, been fought by the consumer with some passion and, if not won, then at least fairly honourably drawn. Free-range eggs, or better (as opposed to battery eggs laid by hens in tiny cages), now account for around 50 per cent of all UK egg sales to the public (though the food industry continues to use vast quantities of battery eggs).

If nothing else, that proves that, when it comes to the way our food is being produced, consumers do have teeth. It's time to sharpen them again, urgently, by chewing on chicken that has lived a half decent life. And by boycotting the kind that you can suck through a straw.

September 2004

Keeping it veal

Let me say straightaway that I believe the crate system of rearing calves for veal is indefensible. The animals are so confined that they can't turn round. All they can do is stand up, lie down and eat their daily dosage of powdered-milk-based liquid feed. Denied any grazing or cereal food, which they would normally begin to have alongside their mothers' milk within a few weeks of birth, the calves' stomachs fail to develop properly.

The object of this system is, above all, to keep the meat as pale as possible: in the end, sheer whiteness, rather than flavour or tenderness, has become the principal marker of 'quality' in Dutch crate-reared veal. As a symbol of human indifference to the suffering of animals, that takes some beating.

But this is not the whole story. What few consumers realise is that to banish veal forever from our shopping list and our menu is to condemn potential veal calves to a heinous fate. If there is no market for veal, then the thousands of dairy calves born each year that are neither suitable for beef production nor needed for replacing the dairy herd will be shot within a few hours of birth and promptly incinerated or fed to foxhounds.

To keep up their milk yield, dairy cows must take a break from producing it and have a new calf every year. So the number of calves born to the dairy cows in this country is staggering – far greater than is necessary to provide replacements for retiring dairy cows, who may be productive for as long as six or seven years. And what will happen to all those male calves, who could not replace a dairy cow even if you wanted them to?

Once upon a time the calves that were unwanted for, or unsuited (by gender) to, milk production would have been milk-fed for four to six months or so and sold as veal. It is an awareness of this practice and the fact that, to a large extent, the dairy industry and the veal industry are one and the same thing, that turns some vegetarians into vegans. Personally, I can only admire such moral consistency. However, the fact is that the production of veal is not intrinsically cruel, any more than the production of pork, beef or lamb is.

Crucially, the age of the animal at slaughter really is not, or should not be, the issue. Veal calves are generally slaughtered at five or six months – precisely the same age range as pigs for pork and sheep for lamb. You may think that is too tender an age to be slaughtering any animal for meat, in which case you should stick to mutton and beef, and try to find someone who keeps pigs to bacon age.

But to make one rule for pigs and sheep and another for cows just does not make sense. I don't want to get into a debate about whether a short life of misery is ethically any more acceptable than no life at all (I happen to think it isn't). But fortunately I don't have to. Because the cruelty of confinement or the shame of execution at birth are not the only alternatives for these animals.

There is a system of veal-calf rearing that is far more extensive than the Dutch crate one. The resulting product, from free-range calves that have lived unconfined, used to be known as 'bobby veal', but is now being marketed as rose veal, in acknowledgement of the pink tinge of its meat – an indication that, as well as enjoying freedom of movement, the calf is also able to ruminate on a diet that includes some roughage.

Calves for rose veal are now being reared under both conventional and organic systems. In the former, calves are weaned from their mothers shortly after birth (like all dairy calves) but are then reared in loose stalls, in large barns open at either end to let in daylight. They live in small groups, with straw bedding and an 'ad lib' diet (accessible at all times) of both milk and cereal-based feed. They can also graze freely on their bedding.

It is an indoor system, without the obvious and desirable benefits of grass underfoot and sunlight overhead. The standard of welfare depends, in the end, on the conscientiousness of the practitioner. But well-maintained indoor housing, with plenty of space, is at least an environment in which a group of calves can thrive and grow, and should not suffer unduly.

At Hill End Farm in the village of Brinkworth, Wiltshire, Joe and Ro Collingborne started producing rose veal at their dairy farm to prevent male dairy calves being shot; the calves now stay with the cow for four to five months and are reared in a large straw-bedded barn.

The organic system of rose veal production, pioneered at Helen Browning's Eastbrook Farm in Bishopstone, Wiltshire, is also based on a loose housing system, supplemented by free access to outdoor grazing on organic pastures during the spring and summer months. The calves are reared with, or rather by, surrogate mothers, or 'nurse cows', which continue to suckle them throughout their five-to-six-month lives. Both mother's milk and the supplementary cereal-based feeds to which they have unrestricted access are, of course, certified organic. Little Warren Farm in East Sussex won the Soil Association's Best Veal award in 2003 for its organic veal produced from calves that suckle their mothers for six months.

I have tried Eastbrook Farm's organic veal and I think it is excellent. The meat is delicately flavoured compared with beef, but it is still robust and tasty. The veal chop that I had grilled with garlic and rosemary was far more interesting to eat than any white veal I have ever tried. And the *osso bucco* was superb.

These commendable ventures provide not just great meat, but one of the most constructive and humane solutions to the particularly challenging ethical problem of redundant dairy calves. I can only hope that other organic meat producers will follow suit, and that you, the consumer, will stimulate the market with your custom so that this high-welfare organic product puts British veal back on the map.

June 2004

Fox in a box

I reckon the old nursery rhyme is at least partly to blame:
A'hunting we will go
A'hunting we will go
We'll catch a fox
And put him in a box
And never let him go!
I mean, it's so cruel, isn't it? Hardly surprising that subconscious guilt, festering in our infancy, rises to the surface and brings so many of us out in favour of the fox.

Of course the rhyme doesn't accurately describe the activity of fox-hunting at all. Putting him in a box, and never letting him go, is much more cruel, obviously, than chasing him with dogs – which will, as pro-hunting campaigners are ready to explain with varying degrees of patience, either fail to catch him altogether, or kill him efficiently within seconds of catching up with him.

Things might have been different if the nursery rhyme had been written about the intensive farming of pigs:

We'll grab a sow
And put her in a box
And never let her go!

At least, not until she's had over 100 piglets and is so worn out she can't stand up on her own. And then she'll go for supermarket sausages.

It doesn't rhyme (unless you're from Wolverhampton, where I understand 'go' rhymes with 'sow') and the extra line at the end puts paid to the scansion. But it does at least, with reasonable accuracy, describe the business of large-scale pork production. And, had it been it part of our nursery culture, then maybe we'd all now be having a sensible debate about reducing the massive institutionalised cruelty in our intensive farming systems. As opposed to this ludicrously uninformed and hate-fuelled row about foxes.

A lot of people I meet seem to think I must be enthusiastically, aggressively pro-hunting – perhaps because I make a TV show which extols (some) of the virtues of country living. I'm not. I can't be that enthusiastic or aggressive about something that I have never been interested in. I don't really get along with horses – either in the field, or on the plate (though donkeys make a nice salami). I did have riding lessons, after school, when I was about eight years old. But they clashed with *Scooby-Doo* and *Blue Peter*, so I got off to a very resentful start. Then I fell off, bruised my ribs, and refused to get back on.

Now the prospect of trying to steer an enormous horse at high speed across ditches and over stone walls fills me with both terror and abhorrence. At the same time I can, from a safe distance, see that it might appeal to some.

What I can't see is how any intelligent person who had stopped to think about it for more than a minute could ever consider the wild fox in more urgent need of legislative protection than the factory-farmed pig. Compared to the poor pig, who stands or lies on concrete (piled with shit), in such close confinement with his hundreds of neighbours that his unnatural inclination is to chew their tails off, the fox is having a whale of a time. Whether he's made his home in the fields and woods, scoffing the squire's pheasants, the baby bunnies, and too many of my chickens, or living it up in the town, feasting on bins and discarded KFCs (in which case I feel sorry for him, but I don't think he feels sorry for himself), he's doing very nicely, thank you.

The fact that, once in a while, he has to run the gauntlet of a pack of braying hounds, and risk a quick, though admittedly gory, death, is undeniably a bummer for him – and highly emotive for the human observer. But why, when many millions of other animals are, in the name of human pleasure and satisfaction, enduring so much more misery, and not merely in death but throughout their entire lives, has the killing of a few thousand foxes become a matter for parliamentary intervention and furious national debate?

It might all begin to make a faint glimmer of sense, an almost forgivable kind of well-intentioned, if misguided, moral zealotry, if even one anti-hunting MP (or one furious hunt saboteur, come to that) was saying, 'We just want to sort out the hunting thing first – it's been bugging us for SO long. Then we'll start looking at the pig situation . . .'

But they're not. Instead they're saying shooting will be next. Then fishing. Here are two pursuits I do enjoy, and I do understand. Not least because they have afforded me some of my finest meals.

My personal view is that when shooting and fishing are seriously under review, the logical absurdity of a legislated ban will become too gross for all but the really stupid, or the really embittered and entrenched, to overlook. I'm certainly prepared to invest a lot of time and energy arguing the point.

I mean, how, sensibly, can you ban fishing with a rod and line on the grounds of cruelty, but not ban commercial gill-netting, by which millions of fish take many hours to slowly twist, exhaust and suffocate themselves to death?

And isn't it blindingly obvious that the lot of any wild bird, and even the half-wild pheasant reared for shooting, is, even if it meets its end by being blown out of the sky with a shotgun, still infinitely better than that of the factory-farmed chicken?

And isn't it most obvious of all that the quality of an animal's whole life, which will be measured in weeks, months and years, will always be of far greater significance in any ethical assessment of welfare and cruelty, than the manner of its death, which will usually be a matter of seconds, or, at worst, minutes.

The problem is, of course, that all manner of cruelty is permissible when animals are being raised and slaughtered for food. It's business, and God forbid that any MP of any party these days be seen to be interfering with that sanctified pursuit. But hang on, aren't hunting, fishing and shooting also businesses? Well, only in the sense that tens of thousands depend on them for their living. I mean they don't actually make anyone seriously rich – at least not in the order of magnitude that might tempt them to make a donation to a political party.

But don't fishing and shooting also provide us with food? Some of the best meat you can hope to lay your hands on? Or is it just a few weirdos like me who think that way?

Relatively speaking, it probably is. But it's becoming ever more clear to me that us weirdos, and the wild meat we insist on making part of our diet, provide one of the last and most vital checks on the relentless intensification of meat production. This is because the mammals and birds we kill with our guns, and the fish we haul out on our hooks, are a vital reminder of where all our meat once came from – and of a natural lifestyle to which we should aspire for all our food animals.

Those factory-farmed pigs and chickens need us – we are their greatest hope of liberation, if only because we remind our fellow diners that all the animals we use for food were once wild and free. And if ever it becomes illegal to acquire meat by the use of a gun, they, and we, are absolutely stuffed.

October 2004

Vegetarians with teeth

'How do you know stegosaurus is a vegetarian?' asked Oscar.

'You can tell from his teeth,' I said, feigning confidence in my hazy paleontological recollection. 'Dinosaur experts think they weren't the right teeth for eating meat.'

'But Ned's got the right teeth for eating meat, and he's a vegetarian too,' said Oscar.

Good point, I thought.

'Well, Ned has a choice, because he's a human being. Animals either are vegetarians, or they're not.'

'I'm a shoe-man bean. Does that mean I can choice?'

'Yes,' I said.

'Well, I'm going to choice to eat meat then.'

'Why's that?' I asked.

'Because I like it.'

'Me too,' I said.

What I didn't say to Oscar is that I have been thinking a fair bit recently about the whole vegetarian/carnivore thing. Why exactly do I eat meat? I don't think it's particularly good for me (partial as I am to the fattier cuts). I abhor the way most of it is produced. And, much as I enjoy eating it, I don't imagine life without it would be completely unbearable. So you see, I am not an untroubled carnivore. So why haven't I become a vegetarian?

Well, I guess there's my image to think of. Connoisseur of obscure body parts. Enthusiastic muncher of small furry animals. But honestly, I'd give it all up – even the bacon – if I was properly convinced it was the right thing to do. Recently, I've been considering the matter in some depth for a book I'm working on. Soon I hope to have resolved the matter to the satisfaction of my own conscience – one way or another.

But in the meantime, there's one thing I'd like a bit of help with. And perhaps there's a vegetarian out there who can oblige. (Or, more likely, a vegan, because what vegans understand, to their credit, is that the dairy industry is the meat industry – or at least the beef industry.)

My questions are these: what would the vegetarian Utopia look like? And would anyone seriously want to live there? How would vegetarians set about dismantling the mixed farming system? What would happen to all the farm animals?

One possible response is that because killing animals is simply wrong, a moral absolute, questions like mine are irrelevant (as well as irritating). But that really isn't good enough. Because if enough of us were genuinely persuaded of the wrongness of killing animals for food (which is presumably what vegetarians would like to happen) we could then choose democratically to live in a meat-free society, and these questions would become very real.

Would vegetarians then be in favour of the mass slaughter of farm animals, to accelerate the arable revolution? And if so, would the carnivorous minority be allowed a last supper of the slaughtered corpses? Presumably the answer is 'no' on both counts.

More likely, the WPTVB (Working Party for the Transition to a Vegetarian Britain) will favour a gradual scaling down of stocking, to a point where small populations of a wide range of breeds are managed, by man, in 'Tame Life Parks'. Here they are well looked after and preserved for their educational and historic interest. Meanwhile the countryside is turned over to the cultivation of fruit and vegetables – grown, of course, without the aid of animal manures, and therefore with the input of huge quantities of chemical fertilisers.

But the matter cannot quite rest there. What happens when the sheep and cows get a bit long in the tooth? Or short in the tooth, as is the problem with ageing livestock. They can't feed properly, and quickly lose condition. In the absence of predators to finish them off, they will die a lingering and stressful death. Will the vegetarians allow human, and humane, intervention? Can we 'put them out of their misery'? And, incidentally, do we then incinerate their carcasses? Feed them to our pets? To the worms? Or, as a sop, to those appalling carnivores, for an occasional 'treat'?

I guess what it boils down to is this. All animals must live some kind of life, and die some kind of death. And having died, they will be eaten, whether it's by a maggot, a crow, a fox . . . or a person.

The carnivore's position, and mine until you persuade me otherwise, is that the best, most morally acceptable way to co-exist with our dependent, domesticated livestock is to take care of them when they are alive, ensure they have a quick and, in relative terms at least, stress-free death. And then eat them.

I accept entirely that, through industrial farming practice, we are guilty of a gross abuse of our responsibility of care, and a treatment of farm animals that is often morally without defence. But surely reform, and not abstinence, is the answer?

If you're a sheep, the question of who ends up eating you when you're dead is the very least of your worries. And, in the long run, you'd probably rather be a sheep than a stegosaurus.

May 2003

And if there's one thing worse than unthinking vegetarians, then it's hypocritical carnivores . . .

It makes me wild

In recent weeks I have been called a pervert, a maniac, a sadist and even a murderer. I have, it seems, upset a few people. What exactly have I done to incur their wrath and their rather unimaginative insults? I have appeared on television and demonstrated the cooking of a few of my favourite recipes – some of which involved meat. Delia Smith has done this. So have Keith Floyd, Sophie Grigson, Ainsley Harriott, and a few dozen others. Have they suffered the same abuse? I suspect not.

So why have I been singled out for attack? It couldn't possibly be, could it, because the meat I chose to cook did not come from the supermarket wrapped in cellophane? Because the animals from which it came were never restricted, restrained or abused in any way, but free-roaming throughout their lives? Because they fed only on a natural diet, selected entirely by themselves? Because they were not injected with any hormones, growth promoters or chemicals of any kind? Or because they were never transported for slaughter, but killed swiftly and humanely in the place where they lived?

Perhaps it's unfair of me not yet to have mentioned the fact that, in many cases, my programmes also showed the capture and even the killing of the animals I went on to cook. And that these animals were not, in the minds of many, those most commonly recognised as food: I killed and cooked in the course of the series crayfish, a hare, some eels, a few zander and some young rooks.

I don't expect everyone to enjoy a programme that takes an interest in traditional methods of trapping and killing animals for food. They can always turn over and watch *Top Gear*. But when they write me letters, or leave irate messages with the Channel 4 duty log, saying they would like to see me fried in oil, or how would I like it if my babies were stolen from me and eaten by a monster, I have to hit back: You hypocrites! You hysterical, blinkered, unthinking hypocrites! Most of you do not even have the consistency or the moral fibre to become vegetarians.

I know this because, of the numerous committed vegetarians of my acquaintance, the majority actually approve of what I do in my programmes, even if they choose not to do it themselves. They understand that even though we choose to fight our battles with different weapons, we have a common enemy: the industrial farming community, who have reduced the art of food production in this country to a mechanised production line of institutionalised inhumanity, where quality counts for nothing and compassion even less.

But what do *you* understand, as you munch your ham sandwich or pick up a Big Mac on the way home? That a squirrel has a fluffy tail, and looks cute when it steals nuts off the bird table. Well, let me tell you, its back legs are as tender and tasty as a partridge, and they cook like a dream on the barbecue.

Don't you realise that everyone who eats meat condones the killing of animals for food? Every time you bite on a cocktail sausage or a BLT you support the mass production and slaughter of an animal that is probably more intelligent than the pampered poodle lying at your feet. Unlike you, who understands nothing about the origins of what you eat, I am prepared to take some trouble to find out where the meat I eat comes from, what the animals have been fed on and how well they have been treated. Unlike you, I am also prepared to take responsibility for the manner of the death of the things I eat. That is why I choose to eat fish, shellfish, birds and animals I have cooked and killed myself. If that makes you uncomfortable, then stop eating meat now. But be careful not to choke on your nut cutlet.

May 1999

The following piece was commissioned for a Sunday supplement, but was never published. The fishing safari company that arranged the trip somehow got hold of it before it ran, and complained that it was 'too negative'. The commissioning editor asked me to make some changes that I didn't agree with. Stalemate ensued.

I wanted to include it here, partly because this trip is a powerful memory for me, but also because it touches on the ethics of fishing. Part of the fun of fishing – and I really do find it fun – is the sensation of doing battle with a struggling fish at the other end of the line. Hence the ultimate fishing experience being the pursuit of the biggest, strongest, fastest fish of all – the marlin. Yet, as you can see, my brief encounter with it left a strange taste in the mouth . . .

Off the hook

'Nothing I can tell you will prepare you for it,' said Gary Cullen, manager of the hotel's fishing operation. 'If it happens, you won't believe what you see.' I was dining with the white Kenyan skippers of the boats, my fellow fishermen, and their wives (who weren't coming) on the hotel veranda overlooking the beach and the bay. As we ate our baked crab, steak and chips, I watched the crew of 'locals' (black Kenyans) loading up a little dinghy with cold-boxes, ferrying out supplies of ice, beer and food to the boats we would be taking. I never heard the Europeans bad-mouthing their African crew, but the old colonial lifestyle is alive and well on the fishing boats of Kenya.

By half-past midnight we were leaving behind the yellow lights of Watamu, with a six-hour journey ahead of us before we reached the fishing grounds. We trailed a garish 'Honolulu' behind the boat – a fluorescent rubber squid almost a foot long, in which was hidden a hook as wide as a hand, with a shank as thick as a six-inch nail. This was 'on the off-chance' – a strike was not expected until the morning. My instructions were 'to try and get some sleep', but they might well have told me to try and walk on water.

For I had come to Kenya to realise every fisherman's wet dream. I was here to catch the biggest, fastest, hardest-fighting fish that anglers ever seek to catch on rod and line: the marlin.

I awoke, not from real sleep but from that restless hinterland of racing thoughts and images, in this case fish-related, to smell breakfast and see the sun was up. After toast, fried eggs and tea, the full set of seven rods was rigged up, and the serious fishing began. The lures are spread apart from each other by 'outriggers' – curving poles which sprout symmetrically from either side of the boat. Line is taken from the tip of the rod, and held by a clip at the end of the outrigger. A striking fish will pull the line from the clip, and then be in direct contact with the rod again. I watched the parallel lines trailing out from the back of the boat, and applied my tired mind to the simple and satisfying thought that now, at last, I was fishing for marlin.

The first excitement was not long coming, though it didn't come to me. One of the other boats, about 500 yards away, radioed to say they'd had a strike. Looking over towards it, I could see the silhouette of a figure in the fighting chair, and just make out the arc of a straining rod. 'What's he got?' I asked. 'Watch,' said somebody. Suddenly, between our boat and theirs, I could see white water; something flashed above the sea, catching the sun. My eyes took a snapshot, and retained an image I can still recall: the fish stood on its tail, curved like a backwards 'C', its silver-white belly flashing like a mirror, the line of its dark back flickering with the sun's gold.

I was the only one who hadn't seen such a sight before, but the others weren't much less awestruck. 'That's what it's all about,' said the skipper, after a short silence. The fish was a striped marlin, the smallest of the three species we could expect to encounter. The blue is bigger, the black the giant that every game-fisherman dreams of catching.

The skipper of the lucky boat radioed to say the fish had been successfully boated, tagged and released. This is a practice recently initiated in the United States by the Oceanographic Institute, as part of a long-term project to study the migratory patterns of bill fish (marlin, sailfish and swordfish) and assess the populations. The individual angler has the choice of killing the fish, or releasing it tagged. The practice is the topic of much heated debate among game-fishermen, some of whom believe that the fish are not capable of surviving the trauma and physical strain of being caught, and inevitably die shortly after being released. The releasing of fish hasn't gone down too well with the Africans either, who see it as an appalling waste of scarce protein.

The knowledge that, should my turn come, a fish's fate would be in my hands, stirred my conscience. The fish I had just seen was, theoretically, swimming free again. Maybe that was a good thing, if it really was going to survive. But to release a fish makes the catching of it an act of the purest vanity. It is as if, in defiance of nature, the fisherman is saying 'Look what I can do, look at the games I can play with your creations'. The hunter can enjoy the hunt, but should never forget why he is a hunter. I decided that I would kill whatever I caught – and insist on eating a piece of it too.

Not that anyone would have urged me to release the first fish that came my way. I had finally managed to doze off when someone shouted 'Outrigger!', and I heard the line screaming off the reel of the rod beside me. I picked up the rod and as I struck hard to set the hook I remember thinking 'It's a marlin but I know I'm going to lose it.' In fact neither of those things were true. When I realised the fish was still on, and started to wind in the line, the skipper said, 'Don't get too excited, it's only a dorado.' Whatever it was wasn't keen to come to the boat, and went off on a second searing run at right angles to our bows. 'It's good eating, mind,' added the skipper, and as if in response to this threat the fish leapt right out of the water, revealing its curious machete-shaped head and its brilliant gold colouring. Eventually it came to the gaff, but not before demanding enough effort from my forearms to make me feel I had just lost an arm wrestle with someone only marginally stronger than I was. The fish was about 15 pounds. 'What we're trying to catch eats that for breakfast,' said the skipper, putting my achievement in perspective.

The rest of the day was punctuated by occasional encounters with dorado, and small tuna. These were fried and eaten, washed down with our cold beers, as the sun was going down. As I savoured the crisply frazzled pieces of indecently fresh fish – a little overdone and a little oversalted, but somehow all the better for that – the skipper explained to me how the night's fishing was going to work. We couldn't expect marlin after dark, but would be drift fishing with real squid, in the hope of picking up a swordfish.

I had been enjoying my first spell of real sleep for 48 hours when voices and an apparently fishy commotion disturbed me. I was summoned to the fighting chair: 'It's not a broadbill, but it's something quite hefty,' said the skipper. It felt like I was winching in a large sack of coal. The only resistance was an occasional weighty tug; there might have been a large dog on the end, shaking the bait occasionally like a favourite slipper. What did appear at the end of the line was hardly less surprising: its tail, body and dorsal fin were clearly those of a shark; but its huge mallet-shaped head might have been grafted on by some undersea Dr Mengele. It was, in fact, a hammerhead shark.

Its apparent indifference at being hauled to the boat ended abruptly when the first mate tried to put a noose round its head. It went berserk. Having wasted no energy coming in, it was ready to do battle at close quarters. Thrashing its head wildly from side to side, it twisted and squirmed its tapering body like a drug-crazed mobster resisting arrest. Eventually the rope was secured behind its swollen head, and lashed to a cleat at the back of the boat. As the rest of us danced about the deck trying to avoid its flailing tail, the mate reached for a large wooden club, and swung it again and again, crashing down between the empty white eyes. It was five blows before he even drew blood, and at least 20 before the wild thrashing calmed to the twitching, writhing death throes of a nervous system giving up the spark of life. This was not the honourable duel between man and fish I had day-dreamed about; it was more like a gangland slaying.

The rest of the night was uninterrupted by fish, and I slept for a few hours. The following morning we again put out our shoal of seven lures, and trailed them through the dead calm waters beneath the blistering sun. On board, chatter gradually faded out and we were left with the unchanging tone of the engine. For several hours we cruised without sighting a fish. 'You can bet a few fish have seen us, though,' said the skipper. 'Sometimes they just won't come up.'

'What can you do?' I asked.

'If we can find some tuna, we could put a live bait on a down-rigger. That sometimes gets them going.'

Ten minutes later we saw a flock of terns ahead, diving into the water after bait-fish. Steering a course through them, we were suddenly in business: within a few seconds, three of the rods were streaming out line. The fish were bonito – small tuna, of only a few pounds. But they gave a good account of themselves, reminding me in no uncertain terms what something higher up the food chain might be capable of. The one I brought in, about ten pounds in weight, was selected as live bait.

Live-baiting is a grisly business, which makes you hope a fish's nervous system is as primitive as biologists tell us. The hook is 'sewn' to the nose of the bait-fish with a baiting needle, the thread being passed through one eye and out of the other. My bonito, stitched up in this way, was thrown back into the water. The down-rigger, a weight of about five pounds on a wire cable, was fixed to the rod-line with a release clip, and winched down to about 30 yards. We trolled the tuna steadily at just a few knots. The brutish reality of this scenario, like tethering a goat for a tiger, made some kind of drama seem inevitable.

When the fish struck, I happened to be sitting in the fighting chair holding the rod. Two or three sharp knocks on the line indicated something was taking an interest.

'Could be a shark too small to take the bait,' I suggested.

'No such thing,' said the skipper, then added 'Be ready.'

I braced myself, but not sufficiently for the force that suddenly pulled me out of the seat, and cracked my knees against the back of the boat. 'Strike now!' shouted the skipper, and I threw all my weight backwards against the force of the charging fish.

'And again!'

With the second strike I staggered backwards, collapsing into the fighting chair, as the line continued to tear off the reel. 'If he's hooked, he would have jumped. Strike again.' I was about to swing the rod back for the third time when I felt the line go slack. Behind the boat, from the middle of the wake, a dark shape erupted skywards, sending spray out like a depth charge. No more than 50 yards from where I sat – it seemed to be looming over me – a huge black fish was airborne, water cascading from its flanks, its bill, like cold blue steel, pointing straight up at the sun. As it fell back into the sea, a violent shake of its head sent something flying upwards, spinning high into the air like a silver boomerang.

It was the bonito live bait, and with it my hook and line, contemptuously eructed by the taunted fish. In stunned silence, I reeled in the slack. 'That was a good-sized black,' said the skipper. 'Maybe 500 pounds,' said the mate. I couldn't speak, for none of my day-dreams had prepared me for the sight of something so huge, beautiful and superior bursting out of the sea. That it might not have got away, that, with better luck, or skill, or strength, I could have brought it beaten to the boat, and killed it, even eaten part of it, now seemed to me impossible.

It was late in the afternoon, the fish was back in its element, and it was time for me to return to mine. The journey back seemed slow and lumbering, now that I had experienced the power and grace of a marlin moving through the water. We had been heading for shore for a couple of hours, without speaking, when the skipper made a resonant remark: 'You realise if it had stayed on the line, you might just be bringing it to the boat about now.'

That would have been an extraordinary two hours. But I can't say for sure I would have enjoyed it.

May 1991

You could say I have 'got over' most of the qualms hinted at in this piece. I still fish with live baits, and I must have knocked many hundreds, if not thousands, of fish on the head, in the 15 years since I wrote this. But as with raising my own livestock and taking it to slaughter myself, I find the catching and killing of fish, far from inuring me to matters of morality in our carnivorous habit, actually help keep such issues in the frame.

Of course, when fish have first names, and are practically pets, the ethics of killing and eating them takes on another dimension . . .

Funeral for a fish

The Bahamas. I have no reason not to think they're lovely, but neither are they islands I've ever thought of going to – the Indian Ocean somehow being more my bag, and indeed my wife's, than the Caribbean. But one afternoon I'm staving off the autumn chill by surfing the internet in search of a New Year break in the sun. After summoning a series of virtual Bounty ads, I unearth details of a house called Slipstream, on Long Island, apparently one of the least developed of the islands. It's actually described on the web page as 'like a tropical River Cottage'. Well, how can I resist that?

Once I get talking to the chap who owns it – an internet entrepreneur who happens to be a fan of the show – he is more than ready to expand on the metaphor. I think he senses my weakness, because he says, 'If you're resourceful, and any good at fishing, you should be able to catch your lunch and dinner every day.' Well, he already has me hooked. 'As for breakfast, just reach over the veranda and grab a papaya. They're growing all around the house.' And that's a clincher for Marie. It takes only 48 hours to persuade our friends Hattie and Jerry that they, and their three kids, should come too.

When expectations are this high the moment of arrival is critical – dangerous even. But within seconds Slipstream has us feeling that our three weeks will, if nothing else, be exceedingly cool, calm and comfortable. From the outside it looks grand and sophisticated in its varying shades of violet and blue – just a little bit Miami. But in fact it is remarkably simple, even crude, in its design: breezeblock walls are broken up with lots of French windows, and the roof is a great semicircle of corrugated aluminium.

There's no air-conditioning, but you don't need it because the open plan, open doors and lofty ceiling somehow conspire to catch any breeze that's going. There's nothing particularly fancy about the kitchen strip on one side of the main living space, but it's big enough and it works. It's clear that any fish I should happen to catch can certainly get cooked. River Cottage by the sea, with coconuts? A tad more glamorous, perhaps, but I'm hardly going to moan about that.

But I haven't been in the house more than 24 hours when I realise I might be in some trouble with my landlord – another familiar feeling from River Cottage days. I've woken up early the first morning and am itching to fish. I have a simple exploratory procedure whenever I arrive at a new and uncharted fishing place that is particularly effective in tropical seas. I take two rods, a big one and a little one, to the beach. I try and catch a little fish, on a little hook, on the little rod. Then I immediately put the little fish on a big hook, on the big rod – and try and catch a big fish.

Slipstream is just yards from the beach, and a man-made promontory of piled up rocks, a kind of makeshift jetty, is the obvious place to fish from. I pinch a little bit of bread on a small hook and dangle it under a tiny float just a few yards from the rocks. Within seconds the float darts under the water, and I pull out a wriggling silver-white fish no bigger than my thumb. I transfer it from the little hook to the big hook, and cast it out with the big rod, as far as I can, where it swims about under a big polystyrene float, in an irresistible 'eat me' kind of way.

I go back to catching the tiddlers, wondering how many of them might make breakfast, and if they might not be just a little small and bony to be palatable. I have three or four of them, swimming in seawater in a Tupperware box I fetched from the kitchen, when suddenly the big rod, propped up against a rock, starts twitching. I grab it, and watch the float being dragged across the water. Then I strike. Twenty yards offshore a bar of silver breaks the surface. I start reeling in, and though the resistance is less than I anticipate there is a series of satisfying tugs and wriggles, as

I bring a relatively small but perfectly formed barracuda to the shore, and land it on the jetty.

I know barracuda are good eating, and although this is only a small one (it must weigh less than three pounds), there is meat on its bones and it'll just about do us for supper. But perhaps it's too small to be worth killing. There must be 'cuda out there 20 times its size. A terrifying, if unlikely, thought crosses my mind. What if it's the only fish of any substance I catch all holiday? I decide I'll show mercy on subsequent small fish, but not on this one. I pick up a stone and knock it terminally on the head.

Back in the kitchen, my son Oscar at least is impressed: 'Look at those teeth!' he enthuses. 'Bit small isn't it?' says Marie.

That afternoon, at siesta time, I take with me to my bed the folder of information about Slipstream thoughtfully put together by Rob and his wife, Claire. One paragraph is particularly interesting: 'The Jetty. The stone jetty, which we hope to complete later in the year, will serve several purposes. As well as providing a mooring for the Slipstream boat, and shelter for the best swimming part of the beach, it will also serve as a small artificial reef, forming a useful nursery habitat for young fish. This is already starting to happen, as you will see if you go snorkelling around the rocks. You may even be lucky enough to see our tame barracuda, Barry, who regularly comes to hunt around the jetty. Don't worry, he's only small!'

Fuck, I'm thinking. He's not only small. He's also dead. The fish in the fridge is, or rather was, my landlord's pet. He even had a name – albeit not a very original one.

Things soon get worse. Jerry, who is a fanatical diver, has spent his siesta reading a book called *Fishes of the Bahamian Reef*. He also has news about barracuda, and it's not good. He comes at me waving this book: 'Here in the Bahamas, a lot of them are poisonous. There's a toxin on the reef, apparently, that goes up through the food chain. When it gets to the main predators, it can be so concentrated it gives you appalling food poisoning. People die every year. And the worst culprit, apparently, is the barracuda.' He puts the book down with an emphatic thud. 'Good old Barry!' he chuckles.

This is great. Not only have I taken the life of a beloved pet but it turns out to have the potential to exact a terrible revenge, and take mine in return. 'Surely,' I remonstrate with Jerry, 'a little fish like that won't have had time to get enough toxin?' 'You're probably right,' he says. 'It says the bigger the fish, the greater the danger. Why don't you eat half, and if you're okay in the morning, we'll eat the other half?'

I ring Darren, a friend of Rob's and our on-island contact and mentor. I tell him we have caught a barracuda and are worried about the whole poisoning thing. He is reassuringly matter of fact. 'The risk is exaggerated,' he says. 'A lot of islanders eat barracuda. And only a few of them get sick. You should be okay.' I don't tell him that I think I have killed Barry.

Everyone else is of the view that the risk, however slim, is not worth taking. But I have already prepared the fish, and made it oven-ready. I did so, with great pride, over breakfast, within minutes of landing the fish. It is in the fridge, with a series of slashes down its sides, into which I have inserted dry bay leaves, slivers of garlic, black pepper, and a squeeze of lime juice. I can't not eat it. It's going to be delicious. Besides, I feel I owe it to Barry to eat him, so that he hasn't died in vain. It has already been decided by Hattie and Marie that the children are not getting any. 'But I want some,' says Oscar, starting to cry.

That afternoon, Jerry, Oscar and I take the boat out to the 'Slipstream Aquarium' – a rock about the size of River Cottage with a couple of caves in it – about half a mile offshore. Here the snorkelling is superb. As well as small snappers and grunts by the hundreds, there are angelfish, triggerfish, parrotfish and even a pair of puffer fish, which obligingly inflate and push out their spines if you pull them gently by the tail. And there is a four-foot nurse shark, which spookily tracks your movements by swimming along the sea floor about 20 feet behind you. This worries Jerry and me, but it doesn't bother Oscar one bit. He is snorkelling in a Floatie and mini-mask, and can see everything that we can, but he seems to be blessed with a curious problem of scale, whereby all the fish look the same size. After our fill of goggling, as the light fades, we put out a couple of lines and catch a few small grunts and snappers.

So barracuda is not the only fish on the menu that first night – nor, amazingly, is it the most popular. 'No, no, after you,' becomes the oh-so-amusing joke of the evening. I manage to dispatch the whole of one side of it, and although I know it's delicious, and keep telling everyone that it tastes remarkably similar to sea bass, I'm somehow not enjoying it. When Jerry starts joking about a curious tingling sensation in the toes, I naturally start to think I can feel one, and I stop eating.

After dinner I feel compelled to call Rob in London, and tell him I have killed and eaten his pet fish. Perhaps I am looking for absolution – confessing my sins and making peace with those I have wronged. Bit late for Barry, I think, as I dial.

'The good news,' I tell Rob, 'is that we have already caught some fish, and they were delicious. The bad news is that I think you may have had a sentimental attachment to one of them . . .'

He guesses at once. 'Not Barry! You've eaten Barry! I don't believe it! You've eaten Barry!' but to my immense relief he is laughing. I tell the story, and as I do my sense is that he minds a little, but he thinks, on balance, that it's funnier than it is sad. His parting words, and I think he means them to sting a little, are: 'Oh, well! There are plenty more barracuda in the sea.' Perhaps as in, 'So why did you have to catch my pet one?'

Barry exacts no revenge. I wake up the next morning feeling right as rain. Or at least as right as is reasonable after several large Mojitos, consumed on the understanding that they might have been my last. But I couldn't be happier to be hungover. It's so much better than being dead. The fact that I have diced with death on day one, and survived, gives an extra frisson to the sense of sheer holiday stretching before us.

November 2003

And this article about Iceland's fishery completes a trio of piscine ponderings:

Scales of justice

I've just returned from four days in Iceland where I went salmon fishing with a group of friends. Arriving at the airport we were told to our astonishment that our entire fishing gear would have to be disinfected – rods, reels, boots and even lures and flies. We had heard something about this practice, but someone in our party had got hold of the idea that it only applied to landing nets, which we thought we were very smart to have left behind. As it was, our entire kit was laid in a long steel trough that had almost certainly been originally designed as a urinal. It was sprayed with a disinfecting liquid and left to marinate in it for a full ten minutes, before being rinsed, wiped dry, and returned.

The whole process only took about 20 minutes, but we all felt it was rather humiliating, as if we had been declared 'unclean fishermen'. In a sense, of course, we had. Iceland cares passionately about fish – more than any other nation perhaps. No less than 65 per cent of the country's GDP comes from fishing. All its coins pay tribute to the importance of this natural resource. Where the rest of the world puts the heads of its political or cultural heroes, or sovereigns or dictators, Iceland puts fish. Cod on the one krona coin, hake on the ten, lumpfish on the hundred. And very beautiful coins they are too. I gave a bunch to my son Oscar, and they earned his deep respect. 'I know why they put fish on the money,' he said to me a few days later.

'Why?' I asked.

'Because you have to pay money to buy fish.'

'Exactly right,' I said.

In fact, the cod is a kind of national hero. One of the few twentieth-century wars to produce an unambiguous, non-Pyrrhic victor was the Icelandic Cod War. They won. We, and the rest of the EU countries, lost. They achieved exclusive fishing rights for a 200-mile zone around their coast. We embarked on the common fisheries policy, and a quota system so profoundly daft that we end up legally obliged to throw millions of pounds' worth of perfectly edible dead fish back into the sea.

No wonder that, faced with the choice between a share of the subsidies, security and trade protectionism of EU membership, and the right to control their own economic destiny almost exclusively through fishing, for the Icelanders there was simply no contest. There still isn't. They enjoy one of the highest standards of living of any country in the world. No matter that a beer costs a fiver a time. Every Icelander I met was always ready to buy a round.

If the disinfecting experience at the airport left a sour taste in my mouth it was soon washed away as I found myself thigh deep in the river Ranga whose icy waters, rippled blue-black like a mackerel's back, slid inexorably through the volcanic tundra. It wasn't long before I caught a salmon – a fat, fresh fish of about 16 pounds, in such rude health that it took me the best part of half an hour to get it to the bank. We didn't kill it. It went into the 'fish bank' – a cage in the river where the best hens are kept for breeding at the end of the season.

It rained hard that night, and all through the next day. As the river rapidly went into full spate, the ice blue turned chocolate brown and became quite unfishable. In the course of that rainy afternoon we sat in the bar of the lodge drinking beer and sipping Schnapps, and our guide Skuli explained how the Icelanders manage their salmon fisheries. One of the problems with the Ranga is that many of the natural spawning grounds have been destroyed – not by pollution, but by volcanic activity. The 'wild' fish stocks now originate almost entirely from man-made fish nurseries in the upper reaches of the rivers. They release the par from the nurseries on just such days as the one we were experiencing – so the coloured waters give the fish maximum cover from predators as they head down to the sea.

We inevitably got around to the subject of salmon farming – and we all had the usual moan about how an industry, one of whose principal justifications should be that it takes the pressure off wild salmon, has turned out to be so greedy, unscrupulous and environmentally reckless that it has actually come close to destroying its natural progenitor. How did Iceland, which itself has a substantial salmon-farming industry, cope with these inevitable tensions? we wondered. The surprising answer was that there barely are any tensions. The brilliantly simple policy that allows the two activities to happily co-exist is that the one is not allowed to happen anywhere near the other – salmon farming is restricted to areas of the coast, mainly the northeast, with a negligible wild salmon run. 'Nobody anywhere has been able to mix the two on the same sites success-fully,' explained Skuli, 'so we don't even try.'

The disinfecting procedure at the airport began to make perfect sense. There may have been no real reason to fear that our fishing tackle carried bugs and diseases that might harm Icelandic salmon. But given the monumental mess we are making of our own fisheries we could hardly blame our hosts for not taking any chances.

As I left the country, my tackle restored to a state of grace by Iceland's pristine water and thriving wild salmon, I somehow wished I could reverse the direction of that disinfecting ritual. I wanted to take some of the good sense of Iceland's long-sighted fishy vision and cast it back into our own myopically murky waters.

October 2003

It's relatively easy – and increasingly appropriate – to become morally indignant about the way we treat, or fail to conserve, the animals we use for food. But when it comes to the business of feeding the world with arable crops, the appropriate points of ethical intervention are far harder to identify.

Increasingly, agriculture is being taken out of the hands of farmers and the communities they feed, and is controlled by huge multi-national businesses – who often wield more wealth and power than some of the countries whose agriculture they seek to control. Genetic modification is at the heart of their programme of global domination. You don't have to be a Luddite to be sceptical of their motives.

Murphy's law of genetic modification

It's been a scary week for those of us who eat food. Anyone who didn't ask themselves whether they had consumed anything containing genetically-modified crops, and wonder, however fleet-ingly, whether it might affect their health, must have either been unconscious (and therefore probably feeding off a drip) or so full of voluntarily consumed sense-modifying narcotics that they, frankly, just didn't care.

The problem, as ever in these cases, is who to believe. There is a bunch of scientists on one side telling us that GM foods are safe. And another bunch on the other side telling us that they may pose all kinds of threats, as yet unknown, both to human health and the environment. But unless we are prepared to delve deeply into the findings of the scientists, and become scientists ourselves, how on earth do we choose between them?

It would be so nice to believe the smiling Mr Blair, as he tells us there is nothing to fear, and happily stuffs another soya-burger down the gullets of the fledgling Blair babes. And so comforting to dismiss the doomsday merchants of Friends of the Earth, who warn of superweeds, and plagues of flu. So what do we plump for, glib or gloom?

I'm afraid to say, I have to go for gloom – and not because I have heard or read any more than the average concerned citizen on the subject. I choose to be fearful of GM, and to heed the warnings of the unknown consequences of its mounting presence in our food, not because I see a tell in Mr Blair's poker face, or because I believe all that comes from the press offices of the environmental crusaders. I do so for two simple reasons – laws of nature and of human nature that do not have to be spelt out because we already know they are true.

The first is often invoked in jest, as Murphy's law: if something can go wrong it will. Applied to food safety issues, and the general business of tampering with nature, Murphy's law is no joke, as the BSE crisis grimly illustrates: start feeding dead animals to other animals, who are supposed to be vegetarians, and sooner or later something weird and unpleasant will happen. The same applies to GM experiments: if it's theoretically possible that GM foods could leap the species barrier and produce superweeds, or inhibit human immune systems, or cause damage to internal organs or foetuses, then sooner or later one or all of these things will happen. Give enough monkeys enough chemistry sets and one of them will blow us all up.

That may not sound very scientific, but then it is not science that is at the root of GM technology. It is the search for profit. And that brings me to the second law of human nature: when scientific endeavour is motivated by greed – man's unnatural appetite to exploit global markets and make millions of dollars – then it is a certainty, not a probability, that corners will be cut, and safety will not always come first.

The science of genetics is waiting for its first major disaster. It may not come for a few years, or even a few decades yet. And it may not be directly linked with GM crops. But come it will, and the companies dealing in GM foods have thrown their hats into the ring, along with the sheep cloners and spare part surgeons, as leading contenders for the prize of 'First Big Cock-up of the Millennium'.

Of course, scientists are just boys with their toys. They will dabble, they will certainly take risks, and we can't really blame them for either. We can, however, blame our politicians, when the sniff of a quick buck leads them to play fast and loose with the nation's health. Tony, it seems, has invited the GM food giants in through the Green Channel without so much as a glance at their passports. He may not actually have been heard to mutter the words 'we'll be your guinea pigs', but you have to assume he did the sign language.

The kind of arrogant display of confidence put on by Tony and his cronies in the last few days is the kind that classically comes before a long, hard fall. It is also of the kind that the louder it is shouted the deeper it is doubted. Right now, the last person I would seek reassurance from on the subject of GM foods is the Prime Minister. He is now so heavily invested in having us believe all is well, that his word on the subject is next to meaningless. It is quite possible that Mr Blair genuinely believes GM foods are safe – only a monster would feed stuff to his kids that he thought might harm them. But somehow I don't think he believes it to be true half as hard as he now wants it to be true.

But safety is only part of the issue. What about openness, information? The statutory labelling policy on GM foods (which is that there is none) is indefensible. I don't care if GM foods are the safest thing in the world. I reserve the right not to eat them unknowingly, just as I reserve the right not to eat saccharin,

MSG and arsenic soufflé with cyanide sauce. Encouraging GM manufacturers to peddle their wares over here is politically inadvisable. Encouraging them to conceal their activities is politically indefensible.

What can the public do? For the time being, and as far as possible, eat organically. At any rate, prefer fresh and frozen 'whole' foods to anything processed and preserved. Assume any processed ready meals, particularly anything containing soya (including 'vegetable oil'), maize (including 'corn syrup') or tomatoes, may be GM contaminated. If you wish to speed up the process of openness and information, boycott stores who do not tell you what you need to know.

The only possible silver lining for this fiasco is that those in the business of honest, traditional food production, and organic farmers in particular, benefit from the consumer's search for complete safety in their weekly shop. That, and the longed-for hope that the public become a little bit more interested in what actually goes into the food they eat, and a little bit more demanding about the level of information the food manufacturers and retailers are prepared to give them.

I am not known for my squeamishness in the face of unusual food offerings, but to GM crops and their derivatives I say 'no thanks'. The truth is, I'd rather eat a guinea pig than be one – provided it hasn't been fed on genetically-modified crops.

June 2000

Why GM will never feed the world

Of course we should be opposed to GM. It is about some of the biggest, richest, most powerful companies on the planet seeking to own and control global agriculture, and who would want to support that? It represents the final theft of the means of food production, away from local, regional and even national communities, into the hands of a few international corporate giants, based in America, who will quickly come to dictate, without opposition or discussion, what kind of seeds and what kind of chemicals will be spread over every cultivatable inch of the world's land surface. And if I overstate fractionally the reach of their capability I fear I exaggerate not one iota the extent of their ambition.

It is utterly, inescapably obvious that we don't need GM in the UK and in Europe. Our agriculture is already over-industrialised and over-productive. We have millions of acres 'set aside' for non-production. What possible benefits could accrue from another step down the road of 'efficiency'? The good news is that most of us are already persuaded by this argument – and by fear of GM safety, of which more in a moment. In Europe, at least, democracy has said no to GM.

The only conceivably acceptable pro-GM argument, that it might help us feed the starving in the poorer parts of the world, turns out to be the most cynical and reckless of all. Far from offering hope and independence to Third World farmers and growers, GM represents the new economic enslavement of the Third World – neo-colonialism by proxy.

Everybody who works at the hard end of the aid business will tell you that it is politics, war, poverty and drought, and most often pernicious combinations of these factors, that conspire to create famine. Which of them precisely can be cured by a genetically-modified seed? I believe they don't yet have one that grows without water, or produces fruits that pacify dictators.

The fact is that if you want to feed the starving, you must dodge bullets, negotiate with warlords, and rebuild infrastructure. If you want to help the starving feed themselves, you must give them ploughshares and irrigation. If you want to help them compete effectively in the global food market place, then give them access to markets and a fair price for the products of their labour.

If, on the other hand, you want to own them and control them and make them mere pawns in your industrial empire, then sell them a strain of genetically-modified seed and a patented production system that means the seed cannot germinate without your additives, cannot grow without your fertilisers, cannot prosper without your weedkillers, and cannot even produce a viable seed for the following year's harvest. You will effectively then own these farmers, and their crops, even to the extent that you will be able to tell them who to sell to and how much for.

Not that GM companies wouldn't go to extreme lengths to convince us of their benign intentions. In one of the most cynical Public Relations exercises of all time, Monsanto are currently flying around the world a group of cotton growers from Africa, who have for several seasons now been participating in a pilot project growing cotton using Monsanto's GM seed. They are giving interviews to the world's media, telling them that GM cotton has increased their productivity, their wealth, and boosted the prosperity and facilities of their community. Yet all this on a pilot project whose success was guaranteed from the outset. Of course Monsanto has the power and wealth to transform a small agricultural community and ensure its short-term prosperity, just as it has the power to give them a fabulous all-expenses-paid trip to charm the world's press. It tells us nothing about their ability to improve the lot of the subsistence farmer and everything about their lack of corporate integrity and cynical opportunism.

So, GM to feed the world? Pull the other one. In fact, the exact reverse is far more likely. A GM dominant agribusiness in the Third World will create the classic preconditions for hunger and famine: firstly ownership of resources will be concentrated in too few hands (this is inherent in farming based on patented products), and secondly the emerging food supply will be based on too few varieties of crops too widely planted. These are the worst possible options for Third World food security. No wonder there is not a single aid agency or famine relief charity that thinks that GM holds significant answers to Third World hunger problems.

But of course, given an almost inexhaustible supply of Western apathy about the plight of the Third World, the above arguments are perhaps less likely to engage the man in the street than the other Big Question about GM. Its safety. So it's worth knowing that here too, large lies are being told by men with remarkably straight faces.

Perhaps the biggest lie is that 'science' has 'proved' GM to be safe. In fact science has done no such thing. The astonishing truth is that science has shown a marked reluctance to undertake any worthwhile investigation of GM safety at all. And the few genuinely independent (i.e. not paid for by GM firms) scientific studies suggest there is much to be concerned about.

Here are a few examples:

Tests on GM Flavr Savr tomatoes resulted in lesions in rats. On a scale of 1–4, severity was scored 2–3, but was described by the company as 'mild' and marketed as safe.

Dr Arpad Pusztai's notorious experiments with GM potatoes and rats showed severe gut problems in the test animals compared to those fed non-GM potatoes. Despite the largely successful attempt to discredit him publicly, Pusztai's paper had been peer reviewed six times prior to publication. Compared to most GM research sponsored by GM companies it remains a model of experimental propriety and credibility.

In GM chicken feed experiments, twice as many chickens fed protein from GM rape (with a PAT gene) died as those fed protein from non-GM rape. The popular GM maize Chardon LL has the same gene, but no safety tests were demanded.

All of the above should make us worry. But the bottom line, of course, is that not nearly enough time has elapsed to be in the least confident in GM safety. Meanwhile, what's the best comparable example that the kind of transgenic tampering that is the essence of GM might eventually lead to some pretty grizzly consequences? Well, for about 30 years there was 'hard scientific evidence' that feeding high levels of animal proteins to grazing ruminants (i.e. dead sheep to live cows) was 'safe', in that no significant health problems seemed to have arisen. Then suddenly, Bingo! We had BSE.

The production of GM foods is in many ways comparable. It involves combining strands of DNA, often animal derived, that could never naturally come together, then introducing these mutant strains to both the animal and human food chain. Such unprecedented and unnatural steps are producing entirely new materials for both the biosphere to contend with on the macro scale, and the human gut to deal with on the micro scale. Why should we be in the least surprised if, at some point, something very nasty happens?

But perhaps the most compelling reason to be against GM is that George Bush and his cronies are all for it. I watched *Newsnight* last night where a shifty-looking character called Allen Johnson, the 'chief US agricultural negotiator', was nervily negotiating a suitably sceptical Paxman. He seemed to think that by ignoring all Paxman's questions, and saying the word 'science' about four times a sentence, he was presenting some kind of credible defence for Bush's unthinking, unblinking support for GM technology and business. Yet he never looked remotely sure of the truth of his own utterances. If this is the man wheeled out to convince us of the safety and nobility of the brave new GM world, then I don't know whether to laugh or cry. I can't help the former, but I fear the latter is the saner response.

June 2003

It is increasingly hard to be shocked by the megalomania of the global business behemoths, or the ambitions of the scarily brilliant men-in-white-coats whose research they fund. But it's not impossible.

The petri-burgers are coming

So they're going to start growing meat in a laboratory. Beef without cows, pork without pigs, chicken without . . . chickens. Animal protein by proxy – muscle tissue from a Petri dish. Apparently, according to 'researchers' from the University of Maryland, it's going to be the answer to the world's food shortage, and the moral dilemmas of meat production and factory farming, all in one blissfully brilliant technological stroke. Is this genius? Does a Nobel Peace Prize beckon?

No! This is moronic! These are short-sighted, power-crazed, intellectually degenerate, self-serving, morally empty imbeciles! They believe they hold in their hands the beginnings of a brave new world of cruelty-free meat. I don't think so. It's more like the final eradication of any vestigial sense of responsibility, or duty of care, to the animals we use for food. Take it to its logical conclusion, and it consigns to oblivion 10,000 years of a relationship that has shaped civilisation – the contract of good husbandry between man and his domesticated livestock.

Now I am the first to admit that that contract is already in crisis, undermined by the inherent cruelty of our factory farming systems. The need to repair it, and restore and rebuild the respect of our own species for the species that we farm and eat, is desperately urgent, both for the sake of their welfare, and our own moral health.

And I can readily appreciate the overwhelming temptation to see an apparent solution offered by this extraordinary technology. It looks frighteningly like a watertight ethical syllogism: you can't be cruel to anything inanimate, i.e. without a central nervous system. Petri-meat will have no such system. Therefore Petri-meat will be cruelty free. It must seem like a no-brainer (if you'll excuse the pun) – especially to those investors and researchers temporarily blinded by the flash of pound signs, and the anticipated blaze of glory (whichever burns the brighter).

But it isn't like that, and it will never be like that. If you accept factory farming against your own stated moral position, as most of us resignedly do when we begin to load up our shopping trolley, and then you accept the technology that promises to replace it, then you also inevitably accept everything in between. After all, who's got time to check up on what these guys are really up to in the lab?

It seems to me far more likely that this Petri-meat technology will never really replace factory farming; it will only ever augment it, in the most grisly, Mengelean way imaginable. After all, another absurdly overfunded group of white coats (with butcher's aprons on top) have already given us the featherless chicken – no plucking required. They are also working on the brainless bird – 'too dumb to suffer', and have pledged to follow up with 'vegetative' versions of pigs, sheep and cows.

From the sound of it, Petri-meat could hardly be more revolting. The researchers are not even beginning to think in terms of anything as sophisticated as a steak, a chop, or even a chicken breast. Theirs will not be meat as we know it. A mass of cells, 'grown' on rubbery sheets of nutrified jelly, it will have no structure, no marbling, no resemblance to a 'cut' we'd ever get from a butcher. By their own admission that is way beyond their technological grasp, and may remain forever out of reach. What they have in mind, apparently, is a bloody, pulpy mush – it sounds like a bad case of roadkill – which will certainly require reshaping, reflavouring and heavy processing.

I see scarcely any conceivable advantage over the dreaded TVP (textured vegetable protein), which has already, in the name of satisfying the sublimated meat-lust of vegetarians, been extruded and flavoured into imitations of everything from a sausage to a lamb chop. But the Maryland team remain convinced that the bovine, porcine, ovine or avian origins of what they can create will give them an edge over anything that can currently be done with a soya bean.

Personally, I would have thought that this will turn out to be reassuringly useless stuff, and so, on balance, I might just about be prepared to sit back and watch this experiment fail catastrophically. Except that I have a deep unease about what divergent paths it might take along the way. What frightens me most is the thought of what might happen when the Petri dish guys and the brainless chicken team get together in a lab and start to party. You know they will. How long before they can 'grow' endless drumsticks on the body of a mutant, anaesthetised chicken? Or create some proteinaceous robo-pig, capable of 'laying' 20-kilo hams like giant eggs?

As long as our farm animals remain whole and natural creatures – identifiable members of distinctive species with a known set of needs and natural behaviours – there can be a reasoned public debate, with hard edges and clear boundaries, about appropriate and inappropriate ways to rear them and take their meat. Consumers can, in theory at least, make their feelings felt in the choices they make at the meat counter. Many of us hope that the burgeoning collective anxiety and suppressed guilt on the part of the meat-eating public may, over the next few years, finally translate into some meaningful consumer action. Things can, and should, get better for farm animals.

But an apparent technological 'fix' to the ethical dilemmas of meat production could spell disaster for farm animal welfare. Under the false promise of moral absolution in their meat-buying habit, the public may be led not merely to accept, but actually applaud, in the name of ethical and scientific progress, a situation where more or less anything goes at the biotechnological end of the meat industry. The thought makes my flesh creep.

September 2005

If you want to opt out of all the scary stuff – GM, E-numbers, agricultural poisons, not to mention systematically abused, chemically altered, genetically abnormal livestock – then the organic label is perhaps the only clear-cut alternative to which you can turn with confidence. That doesn't make the organic movement an instant route to health, happiness, harmony – or world peace. But did it ever say it was?

Missing the point about organics

One of the most popular new themes for lazy journalists – the kind happy to fudge facts for the sake of a quick and zeitgeisty counterblast – seems to be bashing the organic food label.

There's been a flurry of recent articles in both tabloids and broadsheets, 'exposing' the organic movement as some kind of 'scam' because some products which carry the organic label turn out to have a little more salt, sugar or fat in them than similar products which are not organic.

Typically sensationalist and one-sided was the *Daily Mail*'s offering under the banner: 'THE GREAT CON ORGANIC'. The subheading continues: 'Dripping with fat. Packed with sugar. The shocking truth about "healthy" food.' The *Mirror* joined the party with the headline: 'THE ORGANIC FOOD THAT HAS THREE TIMES MORE FAT', and the *Telegraph*, on the same theme, asked 'IS ORGANIC FOOD REALLY WORTH THE MONEY?'

Just how badly can a point be missed? The organic movement has never tried to claim a slice of the weight-watchers' cake, or a bar of the healthy heart chart. Yes, it claims some high ground – both in agricultural ethics and in terms of food quality. But in the former case it merely makes a positive claim for the ecological virtues of farming without chemicals. And in the latter what it principally offers is the reassurance of cereals, fresh fruit and vegetables guaranteed free from chemical residues, and an ethical and natural approach to looking after and feeding the domestic livestock we rear for meat.

In the never-ending debate about taste and flavour, organic producers argue the case for their superiority with only limited success. But they will always be entitled to recognition for setting a benchmark of accuracy and naturalness in the taste of their un-processed commodities. Who can dispute that a beetroot grown in good earth with no chemical fertilisers tastes how a beetroot should? Or that a chicken fed on grain and allowed to roam on grass tastes more truly chickeny than one fed on a refined protein pellet laced with antibiotics and chemical additives, and reared on a litter of its own excrement? These things are true by definition.

Of course a lot of people – sadly it's probably still most of us – don't care one way or another about these issues. But it makes no sense for them to denounce organic farming, or complain about the price of fresh organic produce. It is what it is and it costs what it costs, and you can take it or leave it. You can hardly complain about people who want to produce food uncontaminated by artificial chemicals and additives.

Yet problems seem to arise, and the sceptics and grumblers find the stick with which to beat the whole movement, when basic organic commodities are combined and processed into the familiar 'treat' products of the modern food market place. The consumer clearly wants to have the choice of organic and non-organic cakes, biscuits and fruit cordials, breakfast cereals and jams, flavoured yoghurts and cured and processed meats. Many such products are a commercial success. But is the consumer really entitled to be outraged when some of them turn out, under analysis, not to be a panacea for good health, or an instant answer to disastrous dietary habits?

In the recent organic-bashing articles the selectiveness of the facts and statistics, and cynical spin of the interpretation, varies from predictable and familiar journalistic guile to jaw-dropping dishonesty. For example, there is no question that in many cases, had the researchers not been out to discredit the organic products, they could have found other, non-organic versions of the products under scrutiny that scored worse for fat, salt and sugar than the ones they chose to publish. The worst they were really entitled to say about the organic versions is that they often fall in the normal range for these 'unhealthy' ingredients. And a frustrated and slightly impatient riposte – 'Well, what do you expect? It's a fucking biscuit!' – seems to me entirely in order.

More disingenuous, and sometimes laughable, is the trick of presenting an organic product's undeniable virtue as its avoidable vice. Take the *Mail* article's verdict on vanilla ice cream, organic versus conventional. According to the *Daily Mail* 'the conventional ice cream wins all round. It has half the calories, less than half the fat and less sugar than the organic alternative.' The organic ice cream is being condemned for having a far higher proportion of real (and organic) double cream, and no artificial sweeteners. How mad is that? According to this almost Orwellian way of thinking, a frozen carton of milk would be a better vanilla ice cream than either of them – and an ordinary ice cube would presumably scoop the highest prize of all.

Another gripe is salt levels – fractionally higher in some organic cured meats, and mayonnaise, than in their non-organic counterparts. Of course none of the articles bothers to point out that some organic products may be higher in salt because other preservatives, often made from highly refined chemicals, and including some associated with the risk of cancer and other diseases, are banned under organic production rules. Only 27 artificial additives are permitted under the Soil Association certification scheme, and they are those considered both irreplaceable (by natural alternatives) and safe.

So personally I will be laying on the organics thick this Christmas. I'll be loading my Christmas pudding with organic suet, sugar, flour, eggs, fruit – and booze if I can get it. I'll be basting my organic potatoes with lashings of highly-saturated organic goose fat. And if my home-cured organic ham, baked and glazed with organic brown sugar and mustard, doesn't have more salt, sugar and fat than any of its 'conventional' rivals, I shall consider it a tragic failure.

I produce and buy organic food not to dodge the Grim Reaper, but to celebrate and enjoy my life.

December 2004

We had joy, we had fun, we had seasons in our tums . . . then along came the supermarkets, Permanent Global Summer Time, and the food media revolution. Seasonality is at the heart of the River Cottage experience, and much of my recent writing. I remain convinced that the best thing anyone can do to combat the industrialisation of our diet is to buy more food that is both local and in season. Here's why:

The rhyme and reason of shopping in season

I have just written a book about seasonal cookery. I have done it because I believe passionately that those who shop and cook in harmony with the seasons will get immeasurably more pleasure and satisfaction from their food than those who don't.

I concede, though, that if, like me, you grow your own produce and raise your own livestock, you can hardly fail to appreciate the seasons and their impact on the kitchen. So what about those who don't? The majority who buy all, and grow none, of their food? How relevant is my argument to them? In an age where the transport of food around the world, between the hemispheres and from one climate to another, is increasingly fast and furious, the question inevitably arises: why bother with seasonality? Why not simply embrace the extraordinary array of year-round choice we now have, and cook what we want, when we want?

This is a big question. And it seems that not all high-profile food-lovers share my feelings about what the answer should be. I don't usually single out my food-writing colleagues for criticism by name, but recently I felt inclined to make an exception. Nigella Lawson, who I admire greatly for her book *How to Eat*, last year presented a television series and published a collection of recipes called *Forever Summer*. As usual with Nigella, it was a pretty stunning collection of recipes. But the conceit that ties them together – that, thanks to the wonders of modern farming technology and international food transportation, you can now cook sun-drenched food from far-flung cultures all the year round – really got my goat. It seemed to me both cynical and reckless. As I let slip in a recent interview with the *Big Issue*, my feeling is that she might as well have called the book

Fuck Seasonality. I have just re-read her introduction, and I stand by my choice of words.

In this instance, Nigella is simply the most high-profile perpetrator of a widespread media phenomenon. So much of the way cookery is presented in Britain – in cookery books and colour supplements, and particularly, recently, on television – works against our understanding and appreciation of our seasons. It does so by making someone else's seasonality (or ironically, their relative lack of it) aspirational. It implies that the food and produce of sunnier climes (the Mediterranean in particular) is more worthwhile than our own.

To me this is quite simply wrong. It is a matter of fact, not conjecture, that what is locally seasonal will always be far better than what is not. It's true almost by definition. Most produce doesn't travel well, and the various processes and technologies applied to it to help it travel better are invariably detrimental to its eating qualities. Similarly, the genetic modifications, inputs of chemicals, and artificial light and heat required to grow crops out of season are inevitably at the expense of flavour.

In short, the determination to batter down the natural barriers of food production always has as its motive sheer profit, never the best interests of the consumer. By contrast, seasonal produce, locally grown and locally sold, can always be harvested at its best, and eaten at its best. At my local farm shop you can buy vegetables on the same day they were picked or cut. Cook them (or eat them raw) on that day, before their natural sugars revert to starch, and you will experience a sweetness and acuteness of flavour that you may never have encountered before.

Of course, the biggest culprits are the big supermarkets. They are not merely uninterested in seasonality, but actually keen to suppress it. They have sourced produce throughout the world that homogenises their product range into a consistent, year-long display of cosy familiarity. There is even a buzzword for their mission: permanent global summer time, or PGST. By cherry-picking climates across the hemispheres and around the latitudes they are attempting to create a new agricultural world order, where the sun always shines.

Despite their best efforts, the seasons will still exert some influence on what they stock. Yet they will do everything to disguise this fact in presenting produce to their customers. They fear that seasonally driven marketing will result in inconsistent spending. They don't want their customers to think seasonally, because they believe seasonality is not profitable.

It's a misconceived policy that is damaging to the soul of British cooking. It rests on an assumption that the British food shopper is fundamentally lazy, constantly hankering after somebody else's lifestyle, and irredeemably convinced of the relative dullness of what is local and British.

This is, of course, a circular and self-fulfilling strategy. Reinforce these damning prejudices at every turn of the supermarket aisle and, amazingly, your customers fail to show much of an interest in local seasonal produce. But what might happen if customers were led first and foremost in the store to British produce that is in season, and at its very best, at that precise moment? The supermarket that dares to be different, that celebrates British seasonality and puts it at the heart of its marketing, might just pull ahead of its dull and indistinguishable rivals.

Asda is the first of the big four supermarkets to show some inkling of an interest in such a strategy. A fortnight ago it announced a new initiative, committing itself to putting home-grown produce first in its stores and, perhaps most importantly, to labelling it clearly and unambiguously. The move has been cautiously welcomed by British farmers as about the first piece of good news they've heard from one of the food retail giants in decades. How ironic, and how utterly ridiculous, that Asda will actually have to break the existing labelling laws if it is to keep its promise.

The suppression of seasonality is just the thin end of the wedge. The whole idea of PGST is to present a seamless array of identical-looking produce throughout the year. An extension of the mission to homogenise the seasons is therefore the mission to homogenise the produce itself. One of the best-researched – and scariest – food articles I read last year, was written by Joanna Blythman. She catalogued the numerous ways in which, on the orders of the supermarket giants, farmers at home and abroad are compromising or abandoning the simple quest for good-tasting food in favour of the quest for food that 'behaves itself' in terms of looks, conformity to certain standards in size and shape, and the ability to crop consistently in all the PGST zones.

We are talking about a brave new world of test-tube fruits and vegetables, stripped of the quirks and character that give them interest and charm. To use one of Joanna's examples, the strawberry variety Elsanta, developed in Holland in the sixties, now accounts for more than 85 per cent of the UK market. But it's not a variety you'll find in any fruit enthusiast's garden, or any retail nursery. Because fruit lovers know that it simply has no taste. Its 'qualities' are an ability to withstand weeks in cold storage, then, after artificial ripening by exposure to ethanol, hold its scarlet colour and glossy sheen for further weeks on the supermarket shelf.

These new 'standards' are enforced with totalitarian authority. Farmers unwilling to toe the line are simply shut out of the loop – sent to Siberia, as it were, until their non-conformist commitment to characterful produce is either beaten out of them, or they simply find another way to make a living.

Happily, despite the overwhelming clout of the supermarkets, there are still some small producers dedicated to cultivating the best varieties of our seasonal produce. Increasingly, they sell only through local markets, such as farmers' markets and farm shops. They are the guardians of the vital variations in the taste and texture of produce that allow us, by turns, to be individuals in our own taste. They are our safeguard against a future of bland homogeneity. If we do not use them, we will lose them.

To all who perpetrate and encourage the anti-seasonal, anti-local sentiments about food, be they celebrity cooks, food retailers or the media, I suppose it may be a genuine source of regret that we do not, in this country, have an endless summer. I feel no such pangs. On the contrary, I think we have one of the richest experiences of the seasons of any country on earth. And, shaped by those seasons, and centuries of food production, one of the most beautiful agricultural landscapes too. And we have a range of home-grown produce and a culinary heritage that reflects that experience, and helps to make us who we are. Our weather may be the butt of longstanding jokes among our Continental neighbours, and consequently, in that self-effacing British way, among ourselves. But don't we love it really? Isn't our summer so special precisely because, just like our autumn, our winter and our spring, it doesn't last forever?

May 2003

Here's one that really stirred things up on our website forum, rivercottage.net:

Of pigs and puppies

I took a pig to slaughter this morning. I'll be roasting it on a spit this weekend. It's become an annual event on the farm, which means that each summer I have to select one of my three or four weaners for an early exit. It's a tough choice – one that effectively deprives the victim of another four months of pretty relaxed outdoor living: wallowing in a mud-bath we've made for them, rooting around among the trees at one end of their paddock, basking in the sun, and, twice a day, tucking into a feast of garden and kitchen scraps (broad bean pods and beetroot tops are current favourites).

Last year the decision was made a little easier for me. The day before I was due to cart one off, I went into the run to feed them, and one of them ran straight up and bit me on the knee. 'Tomorrow he'll wish he hadn't done that,' I said to myself, as I hobbled back to the house.

This year I had no such help. I thought I'd try and pick out the fattest one, but they've all done so well I couldn't decide which it was. In the end I made what I guess was a cowardly decision, in other words no decision at all. I simply decided to back up the trailer, throw a few pignuts in, and pull up the tail-gate behind the first unlucky animal that wandered up the ramp. I didn't think I had a favourite, but as the almost-all-black sow with the pink stripe across her right leg nosed her way in front, I realised it was her. But I didn't turn her round. It would have marked a descent into sentimentality.

I didn't mope. I took her up to the abattoir, which thankfully is less than 15 minutes from home – near enough to call ahead and check there's not too much waiting time. Sometimes they'll go into a holding pen for a few hours, but today she walked out of the trailer straight into the slaughter corridor. She walked slowly round the corner, sniffing in curiosity as she went, and less than a minute after she was out of sight I heard the crack of the stun gun. Dead, without so much as a squeal.

I'll be nipping back later today to pick up the offal, and the blood for making black pudding.

They're smart creatures, pigs, and however much I try to stay mindful of the reason I bought them, by admiring their lengthening rack of ribs, sizing up their hams, and wondering what those bean pods might be doing for the flavour of the upcoming roast, it's hard not to be entertained by their antics. I resist sentimentality – but take the view that good husbandry need not exclude the possibility of playtime. On one of those fiery hot days a few weeks back, we hosed them down, and they loved it, snapping at the jet of water like playful puppies. Perhaps that's when I picked out the black one as the biggest 'character'.

I guess that some might take the view that it is easier to be responsible for ending the life of an animal if it is a dull, confined and miserable one, than if it is a fulfilled, free and natural one. All I can say is, not for me it isn't.

Incidentally, I know the puppy simile is accurate, because right now we also happen to have ten of them. Our springer-pointer bitch Dolly popped them out six weeks ago, and you couldn't pick a runt among them. Inexhaustible playmates, they have kept Oscar, and us, entertained for hours every day. Our plan is to keep one as a family pet, and long-term companion for Dolly.

It seems to me somewhat arbitrary though, more or less an accident of culture, that the pig went to slaughter today, while the puppies are earmarked for a decade of pampering and play as family pets. There's no doubt whatever that pigs can make affectionate pets – there are dozens if not hundreds of Vietnamese pot-bellied pigs curling up on suburban sofas all over Britain. They can also be trained in a similar way to dogs. Everyone knows they can hunt for truffles. Less celebrated is their performance as 'gun-pigs' – but apparently in parts of Eastern Europe they were once as popular as dogs for retrieving shot game in dense woodland.

And the edibility of dogs, of course, is as culturally relative as the petability of pigs. It is not the eating of dogs, in eastern cultures, that is barbaric. It is only surely the husbandry – or woeful lack of it – of the canine fatstock, that may rightfully incite moral outrage. Reports suggest that in Korea dogs destined for the pot are treated with extreme cruelty. But for the sake of fairness, we should perhaps imagine our family pets living the life of an intensively farmed pig in a British pig unit. It's no picnic in there either.

So perhaps the time is right for a bit of a cultural experiment. We have already found homes for eight of the nine puppies. With one for us, that leaves one whose fate is still undecided. I say we should keep her for a while longer, and lavish just as much love and affection on her as we do on her sister and mother – not to mention our pampered pigs. We might vary her diet a bit though – plenty of milk, cheese and cereals to help her pile on the pounds. All in all, we shall do everything to ensure she is happy, healthy and gets to do what dogs like to do.

My free-range, outdoor-reared, organic puppy should be oven ready just in time for Christmas.

August 2003

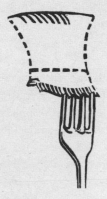

Trends on Toast

**When food gets fashionable,
it should be taken with
a pinch of salt**

So what exactly is the new asparagus?

I was dining recently at a friend's house in London, who had bought some lovely dirty organic carrots from the farmers' market, scrubbed them, peeled them and cut them into batons, and was planning to serve them plain boiled, as an accompaniment to one of his reliably tasty shepherd's pies (no Krug). We were musing on why carrots cut lengthways are intrinsically more appealing than ones cut across, into discs. We decided that there is a one-word answer to this conundrum: school.

This set us off, and as we were reminiscing about the delights of spam fritters, aka Brylcream burgers, frogspawn, aka tapioca, and Pimpled Richard, aka spotted dick, I popped one of the carrot batons in my mouth. Far from getting the light, not-quite-raw-but-pretty-nearly crunch sensation which I was expecting, I found I could crush the slimy thing against the roof of my mouth with only mild pressure from my tongue. The carrots had been, to use a technical term much beloved of top chefs, 'boiled to buggery'.

Partly because Tom is a good cook, and a very good friend, and I felt he could take a bit of constructive criticism, and partly because as a self-confessed kitchen tyrant I am simply unable to keep my food-related opinions to myself, I said to him, casually, and without drawing the attention of his other guests: 'carrots a bit mushy, aren't they?'

'Well, yes,' he replied. 'But haven't you heard? Mushy is the new al dente.'

This struck me as both witty and true enough not to deserve lampooning in *Private Eye*'s new and delightful column, in which perpetrators of this lazy journalistic cliché (according to which something can't be anything worthwhile unless it is the new something else) are held up to ridicule. (The irony is that the Neophiliacs column is, of course, the new Pseuds Corner. Or is it the new Colemanballs?)

Of course, Tom wasn't aware just how true it was. He's not that much of a foodie. He was simply trying to distract from his careless and untypical error by being funny. He didn't know that, by rubbing his mushy carrots through a sieve, and whisking in a knob of butter, and a dash of olive oil, and stealing a little of the mashed potato from under the crust of the shepherd's pie, and mixing that in too to mollify the excessive sweetness of the carrots, and seasoning judiciously with salt, pepper, and just a pinch of mild curry powder, he would create a vegetable side dish that any top toque would be proud to serve, in a rugby-ball shaped quenelle, on the side of his over-sized, over-priced piece of porcelain. Like I said, Tom didn't know that – so I had to do it for him.

Or am I out of touch here? I do live in Dorset after all, and don't make it up to town as often as I used to. Is it possible that vegetable purées of the kind I rustled up with such self-satisfaction in Tom's flat a few weeks ago are in fact, 'so last year!' No doubt you will, good reader, write in and tell me.

The trouble is, of course, that food these days is such a slave to fashion, and fashion moves so fast that even the most loyal slaves are quickly out of a job. It's a knife edge this particular magazine has to walk along every month. *OFM* needs to tell you what's new and exciting and important in the world of food, but not in such a way that it looks like its been taken in by a bunch of noisy chefs who can no more resist a bandwagon than they can a bottle of truffle oil that's past its sell-by date and reduced to clear at £10 a throw.

Incidentally, don't believe any food writer who tries to tell you that purple sprouting broccoli, which comes gloriously into season this month, is the 'new asparagus'. That coveted title, as you see from my list below, goes to the ultra-trendy sea kale – also imminently in season, and coming soon, in a crisp white napkin, to a very expensive restaurant near you. What PSB is, long has been, and always will be, is the poor man's asparagus. That may sound like a less thrilling billing, but believe me, it's ultimately more worthwhile. It's timeless. The poor will be with us forever. The new will soon be the old.

We can only hope, of course, that the 'new-old thing' thing is just a passing fad of a cliché, that will come to be replaced, soon enough, with something, well, newer. So that people will be able to say, 'such and such' [whatever the new phrase is] is the new "new-old thing" thing', and that'll be the last you'll hear of it.

To do you all a favour, and hasten the advent of such a desirable new-old-thing-free state of the language, I thought I'd flog the pernicious cliché, at least in the foodie context, to the point of exhaustion. So there hereby follows an exhaustive list of every edible thing I can possibly think of that is or soon will be the new something else.

And with a bit of luck, that'll be the last you'll hear of this cliché, at least as applied to food, in *OFM* this year – and indeed for ever after.

'Yeah, right!', by the way, is the new 'pigs might fly'.

The new-old foods:

Sea kale is the new asparagus.

Brussel tops are the new greens (it's a Europe thing).

Parsley is the new basil.

Haute Savoie is the new Serrano (which was of course, the old Parma).

Tatsoi is the new mizuna (which is still the new rocket).

Breadsticks are the new-old (i.e. retro) baguettes.

Papardelle is the new ravioli.

Argan (oil) is the new olive (oil).

Mousse is the new ice cream (blame global warming).

Pears are the new apples.

Juice is the new wine (but not for anyone I know).

Varietal Tequilas are the new single malts (but the hangover hasn't changed).

Potatoes are the new tomatoes (astonishing, but true).

Gravy is the new *jus* (as in thick is the new thin).

John Dory is the new sea bass (poor chap).

Fish is the new meat.

Meat is the new bread.

Bread is the new cheese.

Cheese is the new chicken.

Chicken is the new fish (and so *ad infinitum*).

March 2003

I spent much of the nineties being paid to eat in restaurants (please send in your letters of sympathy). The most spoiling aspect of this most spoiling of jobs is, of course, the service – meal after meal where one barely has to raise an arm for the wine bottle. And how do we food critics repay the hours of attention lavished on our comfort and pleasure? By moaning when it's anything less than perfect.

I'd like to take this opportunity to say a collective and all-embracing 'thank you!' and 'forgive me!' to everyone who's ever taken my order, brought or removed my plate, filled my glass or (pre-1999) lit my cigarette. Aside from that, I'll include accounts of just four occasions when I felt inclined, for reasons positive or negative, to draw attention to the service. The first of them was when I was a student pretending to be a restaurant critic. I must admit I find it excruciating to read now. I mean, who did I think I was?

Service game

What is the peculiar disease that afflicts English waiters and waitresses to make them so down-in-the-mouth compared to their Continental counterparts? There are exceptions, of course, but, generally speaking, the English type is reluctant, inefficient, and apparently suffering from pathological disagreeableness. I was served the other day in Alfredo's, one of Oxford's least remarkable pizza-purveying establishments, by a girl who behaved as if she was enduring a sentence of community service for a crime she didn't commit. When I asked her if I could have a side salad, she said 'Yes, but you'll have to pay.' Bare-faced cheek, I thought, to charge for the food, as well as the service.

On the Continent, and thankfully in many of the restaurants run by Continentals over here, waiting is a completely different game. The style varies from immaculate deportment and formal reserve ('Would Monsieur care to see the wine list?' – Le Petit Blanc) to a dazzling display of plate-carrying and bottle-opening skills, accompanied by a passionate speech about Paulo Rossi's goal-scoring ability and Italy's chances in the World Cup (La Cantina).

The Continental philosophy of waiting, which is emulated in all the best restaurants, is that it is an art, not a penance. The unspoken introduction of the true professional communicates a clear message: 'I am a waiter. Allow me to sweep you off your feet with the brilliance of my waiting.' The English equivalent would be something like: 'I am depressed. I don't like this job, and I don't like you. But I have to do it because I'm saving up for therapy.'

Unfortunately the circulation of this magazine is thought to be particularly low amongst the waiting population of the country. So my passionate plea, that present and future waiters and wait-resses should take a leaf out of the Continental book, is liable to go unheeded.

November 1986

Search for the golden crumber

All but the least observant of restaurant goers will have noticed, at one time or another, the various different devices used by waiters to remove breadcrumbs and other unsightly food debris from the tablecloth between courses. Some use dainty little dustpans and brushes; others favour some strange patented plastic contraption not unlike the notorious Remington Fluff-away; still others go for something even more high-tech, with miniature, battery-powered vacuum cleaners. But by far the most common device is a simple bit of low-tech design, with a concave blade in plastic or metal, that allows you to scrape crumbs and other bits to the edge of the table, and into a waiting tray or napkin. I've asked a few waiters what these handy tools are called, and no one can come up with anything more imaginative than 'crumbers'.

Well I've become a bit of a crumber-spotter over the last few weeks, and even asked a few waiters if I can have a closer look at theirs. I've noticed that they come in various different designs and materials, from the bog standard item, which is no more than a handle-less plastic blade, to stainless steel ones with moulded plastic handles, and ones with clips on that allow you to keep it safe in your pocket between crumbing sessions.

A young waiter who served me at Lola's, on Upper Street, had a particularly fine specimen, with a tortoiseshell handle and a silver blade. I'm not sure if it was real tortoiseshell, or real silver, but it looked pretty nifty. He said he'd been given it as a present by the last maître d' he worked for.

The encounter set me wondering: which waiter is wielding the most swanky crumber in London? Are there any in gold, or encrusted with jewels, or made by Aspreys? Are there any crumber collectors out there? I am offering a small prize, which I haven't thought of yet, to whoever leads me to Britain's finest crumber.

July 1997

Dear eau dear

How is it that so many restaurants, decent places where they will take the trouble to ask me how I like my steak, my liver, and my lamb, can make such a mess of things when it comes to serving a simple glass of water? If us punters are prepared to go along with the idea that a bottle of the stuff from the Alps, the Highlands or some Nordic cave is worth £3 more than what comes out of the tap (and it seems we are), then how can you possibly justify contaminating the precious liquid with ice cubes (presumably made of tap water) and a highly scented slice of lemon, without first consulting the person who is going to drink it? It's like serving a glass of vintage Krug hot with a sugar lump and a stick of cinnamon: there's always a chance someone might like it, but it's not what the drink was designed for.

So why the ubiquitous reluctance to simply ask first? Perhaps the practice is now so widespread that waiters are frightened the question will elicit some sarcastic response – like the city suit I once stood next to in a pub who, asked if he wanted ice and lemon in his gin and tonic, replied curtly, 'No, I want it deep fried in batter with salt and vinegar.' The water carrier should not fear such sarcasm. A gin and tonic is a classic British cocktail which, when made properly, always contains ice and lemon. The whole point of a glass of water is that it is not a cocktail. It is the diner's retreat to neutral refreshment: the ultimate palate cleanser. Ideally it should be served cool (at about 4–8°C) and neat, the only essential options being 'still or sparkling?'. If you want to ask me whether I would like ice and lemon – or orange, lime, mango, mint or angostura bitters come to that – I will thank you for your amusing suggestion, and for having the decency to ask. But I will always decline the offer.

July 1997

Oh solo me-o!

The British don't often eat out alone. But when they do, they always take a newspaper with them, or a book. They rarely look up from it, but if they should happen to catch somebody's eye, they will probably scowl. 'Don't judge me,' says the scowl, 'it's not that I have no friends. I'm alone because I want to be alone.'

These grumpy loners will be treated by the staff with a uniquely British mixture of suspicion, contempt, and grudging obsequiousness. This is because no one is quite sure whether they are spies, social outcasts, or – just possibly – food guide inspectors. The whole lone dining thing, though it barely amounts to a social phenomenon in this country, nevertheless makes all those involved just a tad uncomfortable.

In the restaurants of France and Italy, by contrast, from the humblest lorry drivers' café to the grandest Michelin-starred dining room, you will encounter many lone diners. The only thing they will read is their menu, and perhaps the label on their bottle of wine. While waiting for their food, they will sit back, and contemplate the scene. If you catch their eye you are likely to get a smile and a nod – firm acknowledgement of your shared interest in the chef's art. The staff will treat them like kings. This is not because they are suspected of being food critics or guide inspectors but because whoever they are and whatever they do is unimportant. They are hungry, and must be fed. They enjoy good food and must be properly looked after.

I received just such a king's welcome when I lunched alone at Bacco, a new Italian restaurant in South Kensington. I had, of course, taken a newspaper as defence. But I didn't read it. This was not only because it was the *Evening Standard**, and therefore had nothing in it to read, but also because I was so promptly and hospitably waited upon, and my custom was so sincerely appreciated, that I had no need to hide. It goes without saying that this restaurant is managed and staffed by real live Italians.

And I would guess the food is cooked by Italians, too. Artichoke and mushroom soup with croutons is an inadequate translation for my excellent *zuppa di carciofi e fungi con crostini*. A light stock, finished with cream, was strongly impregnated with fungal flavour, and generously swimming with sliced mushrooms, toasted pieces of Tuscan bread, and bits of globe artichoke. Each encounter with the latter shocked the palate with the mildly astringent, nutty-but-soapy taste of this edible thistle.

Harmony was quickly restored with a couple of slurps of the creamy broth. That's another thing about eating alone. You can pay very close attention to what's happening in your mouth.

---

* *An open-and-shut case of biting the hand that was later to feed me. Six years later I was given my own column on the* Evening Standard.

Straccetti di manzo alla rucola e radicchio (my main course) were strips of steak which had been beaten flat, probably flame fried (i.e. flambéed), then served with an accompaniment of radicchio and roquette, which seemed to have been braised in the juices of the meat and a little red wine. That would be my diagnosis, anyhow. However it was done, it was done well, the bitterness of the radicchio and the tang of the roquette enlivening the hot piece of tender meat.

I wasn't sure if I should have a pudding, but with no one to talk me out of it I was unable to resist the sound of *ricotta alla castagna* – ricotta cheese beaten with puréed chestnut, served very cold. 'An excellent choice,' said my waiter. This normally irritates me, firstly because it is usually an insincere piece of flattery, secondly because it implies that other choices I might have made would be less excellent, which makes the restaurant look silly. However, on this occasion I didn't mind. As I was on my own, there was no other person whom he might have thought that I wanted to impress. By this stage of the meal, I knew him well enough to know that he knew that I really would enjoy the dish. And he knew that I knew that he knew. That's how good a time we were having.

As for the *ricotta alla castagna*, it was creamy, nut-jammy, sensual, indulgent – and I chased every molecule eagerly around my mouth with my tongue, without the impediment to my pleasure of a dining companion saying 'Hugh, for God's sake, people are staring!'. And even though I say it myself, it really was an excellent choice.

April 1991

Perhaps what most defined our restaurant culture from the mid-eighties onwards was the relentless pursuit of (and after two decades of media abuse the word is now wince-inducing) 'concept'. This meant the chef, and/or his backers, expressed themselves not merely through food, but also through architecture, décor, uniform, graphic design and even mission statements. This wasn't necessarily a bad thing. In fact, when it was done well, it could make for a truly unforgettable experience – as some of my reviews that follow attempt to describe. But when it was bad, well, it was horrid . . .

Bum deals

The most enduring restaurant concept of the eighties must be the American-style, burger-plus eatery. It comes in many shapes and sizes: there are chains, such as Maxwell's, Sweeney Todd's, TGI Friday, Tootsies and Henry J. Bean's; and there are individual enterprises, such as Coconut Grove (W1) The Rock Island Diner (Piccadilly) and the Dug Out (Leicester Square). Each would no doubt claim to offer something different from the others. And indeed, the 'plus' in the burger-plus formula does vary a bit. With Sweeney Todd's it's pizzas. Henry J. Bean's, on the other hand, has a few Tex Mex options thrown in, as do Tootsies and TGI's and the Dug Out. And the Rock Island Diner. Come to think of it, Sweeney Todd's does too.

One person smart enough to pick up the formula, and endorse it with his well-known name, is furniture-making royal David Linley. His Chelsea harbour restaurant, Deals, has been a great success. So much so, that a replicated version, Deals West, has now been fitted out in Foubert's Place, Soho. I went there to discover what, if anything, the Deals deal has that the others haven't.

Encouragingly, the Linley version of the formula includes a 'Pacific Rim' dimension. Commercially, this has to be a good move. Thai and Malaysian food has just begun to receive the mass attention long given to Chinese. You can even get satay sticks as a supermarket ready meal. Needless to say, it features on Deals's list of starters. Carron (whom you may have met before) chose it in chicken with a peanut sauce. She decided that neither chicken nor sauce compare favourably with the M&S version – and she should know. The peanut lacked pep, and seemed little more than diluted Sun-Pat. The chicken itself had apparently evaded the marinade.

My Tong's yum soup (joke: the chef's first name is Tong) was a version of the classic Thai hot and sour clear broth. This dish further illustrated the danger of offering dishes that are stolen from an alien cuisine. You promise more than you can deliver. In any decent version I would expect to find whole leaves of fresh coriander and pieces of lemon grass. Instead, floating on top were four grubby looking button mushrooms and, worse still, four wedges of tomato. Why?

I followed with one of the cook-your-own dishes – strips of raw marinated beef and my own hot rock to cook it on. This was at least a bit of fun. And one of the four sauces I had a go with – the chilli – was vaguely worthwhile. The other three were so dull I've forgotten what they were. Carron, meanwhile, was equally un-excited by her straightforward steak, served with a range of unrewarding, unoriginal relishes – something sweet, something bland and something else.

It's not that any of our food was completely disgusting. It didn't make us want to vomit – except perhaps with sheer boredom. What depressed us was the feeling that Deals West, like so many other restaurants of its kind, was content to be merely adequate, to keep your average punter, with average nineties' tastes, averagely happy, for an average price. I haven't even mentioned the puddings. They were average.

The fact is, all these restaurants are far more startling for their similarities than their differences. They are all places in which bland food, cheap drink, superficial 'concept' decor and loud music are blended together to make an easy-to-swallow cocktail. The formula has spread from London all around the country, so that there is now at least one restaurant in practically every town about which the following statements will all be true:

1) There are propeller fans on the ceiling.

2) There are old enamel advertising signs on the walls. At least one is for cocoa.

3) The menu is laminated and has what pass for jokes on it.

4) At least four of the following are on the menu: deep-fried mushrooms, garlic king prawns, barbecued spare ribs, chilli con carne, spicy chicken wings, potato skins.

5) The same mediocre chocolate fudge cake is described by one of the following words: outrage, orgasm, heaven, death, oblivion. (How long before someone cuts to the chase and calls it chocolate fuck cake?)

6) There is an extensive cocktail menu – again, laminated.

7) The cocktails are not strong enough.

8) At least one waiter has a pony tail.

9) At least two waitresses are Australian.

10) The bill comes with mints (which, as we now know, will have nine different pee samples on them).

That was all okay for the eighties (except for the pee, which we didn't know about then), when the American way of doing things really was an improvement on our own. The formula is probably good for a few years yet. But the FIQ (Food Intelligence Quotient) of the average British punter is on the up. Sooner or later, the bubble will burst. I can hardly wait.

December 1990

When fish meets fashion

Restaurants with high concepts and mission statements should, in my experience, be approached with some caution. They may shine brightly at first, sustaining the in-crowd for a few months or even a year or two with their glossy package of slick architecture and funked-up menu. But, as we all know, when the Emperor's New Clothes are revealed for what they are, he's not such a pretty sight. His New Menu can lose its savour equally rapidly.

Thus places like Quaglino's, Wagamama and Mash no longer have the cachet of round the block street queues, or waiting lists to rival those for hip replacements. This is because, lined up alongside the competition, including their own imitators, these one-time originals are too often found wanting where it matters most – on the plate. Some of them had it and lost it, others only ever looked as though they had it. The net result is the same: the food lover bolts for the door, with the fashion victim hot on his heels.

It was with this healthily sceptical outlook that I approached Fish! which must be, with its glass and steel housing, its own press release printed on the back of its paper place mat menu, and its unfortunate exclamation mark (how much cooler it would have been to understate that delectable monosyllable), the highest new concept in town.

I went with a friend of mine, Tom, who is a furniture designer by trade and also likes his fish (ideally battered and smothered in malt vinegar). Tom was 'blown away' by the style of the place, and I must admit I was more or less 'knocked out' myself. Tom admired the woven-steel chairs and the cutlery, which he surmised were both Italian. I liked the bar-seating arrangement (Fish! calls itself a Diner), which stretched for a good 30 metres in front of the open kitchen, affording the customer an unrivalled opportunity to scrutinise the food preparation. Having had a quick gawp, Tom and I went to sit at a 'normal' table beside the restaurant's enormous glass wall.

The concept is made explicit on the menu, which, on the back, outlines the restaurant's extremely right-on fish buying policy, viz.: 'Wherever possible we buy line-caught fish' and 'we have asked a team of independent experts to monitor all our suppliers' etc. etc. It also tells you in no uncertain terms that fish is the best thing, healthwise, since Popeye's spinach. This is all, without a doubt, a very good thing, as fish need all the help they can get these days. But all this swanking about quality of supply and joy of fish on the back of the menu puts a lot of extra pressure on the front: it had better be good.

When it comes to ordering there is more concept to contend with: a section of the menu called 'Choose your own' (what else do you do on a menu?) lists over 20 different fish, with little square tick boxes next to each. Those that are available (in this case seven species) have their boxes ticked. I liked this approach, even if it is a bit gimmicky. It emphasises (as if you hadn't got the message from the back of the menu), that everything is market fresh. Or, as I would have advised them to put it if they'd hired me to do their PR: 'if it ain't in good nick, it don't get no tick'.

For our starters we went to another bit of the menu, called 'piscivore', both opting for timeless classics. My marinated herrings were good but not great: the fish itself was unfaultable, but came over-smothered in a mustardy sauce that, while not totally unpleasant, had an over-emulsified, almost bottled consistency. Considering how easy it is to knock up a lovely sauce for herrings from crème fraîche, a bit of English mustard, a pinch of brown sugar, a splash of wine vinegar and a handful of chopped fresh dill, this was a disappointment. Tom's prawn cocktail, by contrast, was exemplary: fat cold water prawns on a bed of shredded lettuce, and a pink sauce that had the balance of ketchup and mayo just right. For my taste, an extra pinch of cayenne and an extra squeeze of lemon would have made it perfect, but Tom was more than happy.

Tom forsook the option of fish and chips with mushy peas, which would have been a good test of the kitchen, for fish pie, which was perhaps an even better one. Topped with creamy mash, nicely browned on top, the fishy bit below boasted a range of species, all worthy of a tick, plus prawns, in a nicely balanced sauce, quite winey and herby and not too milky or floury. It was right up there with the fish pie my mother used to make (she's not dead yet, so quite why she's stopped I don't know) and that's high praise indeed.

But what really stood out, what made the height of the concept and the breadth of the boasting all worthwhile, was my main course: a piece of swordfish, simply grilled, which came with a mild salsa (my selection from a choice of accompaniments, applicable to any of the fish, which included hollandaise, herb butter and red wine fish gravy). I hardly noticed the salsa, because the swordfish itself was so utterly fine. This is a fish which is very, very good when it's good, but so much more often is horrid. A day too long in the fridge or a minute too long on the grill and you have a fibrous juiceless piece of dried up mealy pap. Get it right, as here, and you have the ultimate trade off between white and oily fish: delicate richness, meaty succulence, robust subtlety. This was the best piece of swordfish I have ever had in this country.

If this quality of raw materials and timing in the kitchen extends to the rest of Fish!'s menu (and with swordfish being such a tough one to get right there's no reason to doubt it does), then the high concept swagger seems more than justified. I'd want to go back to be absolutely sure. But the fact that I can hardly wait to do so should tell you all you need to know for now.

March 1999

The Eagle has landed

If I was going to take money off the public for the privilege of sampling my cooking, I would definitely do it in a pub. There are important reasons for this, both psychological and financial. Psychological first.

I can't speak for everyone, but whenever I find myself eating in a pub it's usually because raging hunger has overcome the judgement of a discriminating palate. The safest option is often a single enormous sausage and a side order of disintegrating baked beans. On the rare occasions when you stumble on a pub whose 'chef' has qualifications beyond O-level microwaving, the surprise is so pleasant that you are guaranteed a feel-good eating experience that few established restaurants can match. The option of drinking properly – pulled pints with your meal – is an added bonus.

Financially speaking, the pub offers a chef-proprietor an extremely good deal. If your pub is owned by a brewery, your lease is going to be a laughable fraction of what you would pay for a prime restaurant site in the same area. You can serve drinks, even wines and spirits, to people who aren't eating. And in many cases you can live on the premises – with luck, in a bit of style.

These factors explain the smiles on the faces of Mike Belben and David Eyre, who jointly lease, run, live in and cook at the Eagle pub on Farringdon Road. 'We're on such a good deal it's a joke,' David told me. 'Anyone who is shelling out £200,000 a year for a prime City restaurant site must be crazy.' I don't know if they're laughing all the way to the bank, but they can certainly afford to get there in a cab.

The value-for-money deal on their premises is happily reflected in the prices they charge for their hearty, rustic, Italian-orientated menu. The charcoal grill is applied to spicy sausages, T-bone steaks, fresh sardines and the right sort of vegetables. There's always a hearty soup, such as garlic and cannellini bean or roast pepper and tomato, and plenty of fashionable rabbit food for those who don't want to fall asleep straight after eating. Two courses will rarely cost you more, and often a fair bit less, than a tenner. Why aren't there more pubs in London – and indeed all over Britain – doing this?

September 1990

Well, now, of course, there are. Dozens of really rather good ones, and probably hundreds of middling to mediocre ones too. As the original and arguably best ever gastro-pub, The Eagle has made a fantastic contribution to Britain's dining out culture. Some sort of a plaque would be in order.

'Waiter, are the acronyms fresh?'

If you said you wanted to hit the next food writer who claimed to have discerned a new trend on the restaurant scene, I would have to sympathise. So let me make it perfectly clear that the pattern I am about to describe is definitely not a trend. It is a phenomenon, okay?

We could call it 'Too Many Chefs', but we would probably be in breach of copyright of a new cookery game show format. A description more worthy of the new academic discipline that is post-modern, gastro-sociology would be the Culinary Expectation Gulf Paradox. CEGP for short.

The theory behind this is that the pleasure derived from dining out decreases in direct proportion to the rising standards of restaurant food generally. Or, put more bluntly, as restaurant food gets better, punters are having a worse time in restaurants.

It seems to be a paradox, but I honestly believe it to be true. I'll explain why. Firstly, a brief and grossly simplified recent history of British restaurant food (upper echelon). At the beginning of the eighties there were five chefs: two Roux brothers, a Mosimann, a Blanc and a Ladenis. Between them they taught dozens of young chefs how to cook serious, modern, mainly French, food. A clutch of their protégés became the next generation of stars (the names White, Novelli and Ramsay spring to mind). This second generation has itself now spawned a third, even fourth generation of protégés. Result: there are now probably close to 200 chefs running British restaurant kitchens who can trace their tutelage, directly or indirectly, back to the Big Five.

On the plus side, this means that the standards are higher than ever: incompetence and poor quality are simply not tolerated. On the minus side, this family tree has spawned what may be described (again paradoxically) as a mediocrity of excellence.

By this I mean a large number of restaurants producing food of an undeniably high standard which nevertheless, when experienced on a regular basis, tends towards uninspiring homogeneity. And these are restaurants (there must be 50 in London now) which consider £100 for two a low-to-average spend.

The net result is an increasing clientele of sensation-seeking foodies with sadly jaded palates. Let them loose on the current food scene and, hey presto: the Culinary Expectation Gulf Paradox. Each meal out, in some highly hyped new venue, begins with expectations which are rarely matched.

This is, I think, a phenomenon which top chefs are beginning to sense, and fear. The effect on their cooking is predictable. In their excessive zeal for novelty and excitement, chefs have been producing plates overloaded with the dubious fruits of their hyperactive imaginations.

Anyway, I was musing on this theory of mine, in a mildly self-congratulatory way, as I headed off to dine at L'Oranger. I had heard good things about the food, and read that the chef, Kamel Benamar, was a protégé of both Gordon Ramsay and, previously, the Roux brothers. Surely his food at L'Oranger would illustrate my point most neatly?

How disappointed I was to be. As a theorist, you understand, not as a diner. Benamar's menu is characterised by a refreshing simplicity. Starters are largely classic in form – a soup, a salad, a tartlet, a terrine – with twists that are more tasteful than boastful. My starter of cured fillet of mackerel with a tomato vinaigrette was unimprovable – the fish sweet, suggesting the gravad-style cure had hit it when it was still superfresh, and the tomato cutting it nicely. I can't remember when I last had a starter in a restaurant of this calibre that comprised only two elements. Marie had a salt cod and potato tartlet, a pleasantly peasanty affair, made greedy with a touch of cream, and offset with a *concasse* of fresh chopped tomatoes and shallots.

Main course fishes and meats arrive with fresh seasonal vegetables, imaginatively but not over-elaborately prepared. There is the odd wrapping and stuffing, but most of the meat and fish stand un-adulterated. In choosing a fillet of her favourite fish, John Dory, Marie risked repetition as it came with 'crushed potato and tomato'. But the fish was spot on, the potato and tomato a lovely, garlicky exercise in homey Provençal comfort. I had what may have been the most 'processed' main course: Braised pig's cheek, shredded, and wrapped, faggot-style, in caul fat. It was the least successful dish, but I still enjoyed it.

Even at dessert, the temptation to embellish has been stoutly resisted; the raspberry *sablé* with vanilla ice cream was simple and well done – no mint leaf, no piped chocolate squiggles, no sugar cage.

So does L'Oranger put paid to my theory? Certainly not. It is, of course, the exception that proves it. But more importantly, it points a way forward, out of the quagmire of over-elaboration. The future of gastronomic excellence is the Rigorous Omission of the Extraneous. That's ROE for short.

August 1999

A good omen for Damien

Anyone who ever lived in or around Notting Hill Gate in the seventies or eighties will remember the Cleopatra Taverna, just opposite Hillgate Street, as something of a landmark. With its silver arches and permanently drawn curtains, it had an air of impenetrable seediness and mystery; was it a brothel, an opium den, or a meeting place for Greek gangsters? Since nobody I knew had ever actually ventured inside (the food was rumoured to be awful) such idle speculation could run unchecked for years.

Eventually, when my stint as a barman at the restaurant 192 came to an end in 1988, I decided it was time to get to the bottom of the Cleopatra mystery, and booked a table there by way of a small leaving do. I was promised mixed mezze, half a bottle of retsina per person, plus cabaret – all for just £14.50 per head.

It was an unforgettable evening. I finally confessed my feelings to the waitress I had a crush on, who gently rebuffed me with the information that she was a lesbian. Later in the evening she got so drunk that she slumped over the table and set fire to her hair on the floating candle. We put it out with several glasses of retsina – the heady aroma of pine resin mixed with burnt hair is one I hope never to encounter again.

After a grisly cabaret of bazouki and wobbling cellulite, the band played on and I ended up dancing on the stage with my singed, unrequited love. She spun me round so fast that I finally flew off the end of the stage, and landed, full toss as it were, in the middle of a large table, around which an extended Greek family were still tucking into their mezze. The table collapsed and I was, briefly, knocked unconscious. It says something for the staff that, far from throwing me out, they pampered me and nursed me back to a state where I was sufficiently recovered to order two bottles of Metaxa – one for us, and one for the family whose dinner I had interrupted.

I hadn't revisited the scene of this youthful folly until last week, when I walked into what is now London's most talked about restaurant, bar none. I went to the Pharmacy for a late weekday lunch – which is probably anybody's best chance of getting a table at less than three weeks' notice.

It is no great surprise that the sneering has already started. Damien Hirst's glass walls and cabinets full of pharmaceuticals have (appropriately enough you might think) been getting up some people's noses. I thought they looked fab. I also thought, if I may be allowed a brief stab at art criticism, that the juxtaposition of the ultimate in synthetic manmade consumables with a menu that clearly takes the sourcing and provenance of untampered-with produce very seriously, is both provocative and worthwhile. Besides which, the upstairs dining room, airy, roomy, bright, with a great glass wall view over the street below, is one of the most pleasant I have sat in for some time. And the butterflies in glass cabinets are quite beautiful.

And what of the food? Well, I've read and heard a few moans about that as well, so I arrived with my critical faculties barbed and sharpened. Before we got to grips with the menu proper we had a couple of kirs, and shared, by way of an *amuse-gueule*, a Welsh rarebit from the downstairs snack menu – where everything, as you may have heard, comes on toast. This was a proper rarebit, made as it should by mixing a strong farmhouse cheddar with a little bechamel, beer, Worcestershire sauce and mustard. It came hot and bubbling straight from the grill, and we both loved it.

My friend Belinda started 'real lunch' with a tian of Dorset crab. It was composed of accurately cooked sweet white meat, well- (and not over-) dressed with a loose mayonnaise that had a little pep in it – perhaps Tabasco, perhaps Cayenne. Very nice, as far as it went – though I'm always a bit irritated when you don't get any brown meat on a plate of crab.

My own first course was a wholly successful variation of a favourite dish of mine: mushrooms on toast with a poached egg on top (although on the menu it was rather misleadingly described as 'en croute'– which doesn't mean 'on a crouton'). The mushrooms were wild and an impressive selection – mousserons, *girolles* and *trompettes de mort* among them – for the time of year, and if some of them had been dried and reconstituted it had been done with some skill. The poached egg was a bullet-shaped beauty, judged to perfection, and the whole plate was made a bit lux with a drizzle of heavily reduced wine-flavoured meat juices. In short, a dish that presented a number of opportunities for error – soggy toast, watery mushrooms, badly timed egg – was spot on.

Main courses were mostly familiar combinations without any pretentious razzmatazz – the kind of things that are awful if they are not done right. So my roast suckling pig came simply with a few rounds of fried apple slices. The meat was perfectly tender, not dry, and nicely porky; most importantly, the crackling crackled. The apples were tart and kept their shape (Granny Smiths I would guess), so did their job. The gravy had plenty of porky depth, but might have benefited from a touch of sweetness to balance the apple. Meanwhile Belinda had slow cooked shank of lamb, which flaked unctuously from the bone, and came with cannellini beans that were so soft and creamy I suspect they came from a tin – in which case, I'd like to know the brand.

For afters, Belinda was defeated by an enormous *île flottante*, but I managed every last scrap of a coffee mousse, rich, real and reassuringly undecaffeinated in flavour, sandwiched between some precariously thin and nutty tuiles. Then I polished off the sea of delicious, vanilla-flecked *crème anglaise* that Belinda's partially eroded island was floating in. Then I ate the island.

The Pharmacy may have sent home a few unhappy customers in its first few weeks, but we were not among them. The fact is, you can tell there's a kitchen here that knows about good food, and that is quite capable of ironing out any wrinkles.

Only one thing disappointed me: the men's urinal. Behind the glass splashback (if that's the right word for the place onto which we men are encouraged to pee) is a lively collage of discarded hospital waste: surgeon's gloves, paper towels, plasters, syringes etc. Trouble is, it isn't waste at all. Everything in it is pristine, clean and new. Surely there's room in there for a bit of Hirst blood and pus, something to stir it up a bit? With food this good, the Pharmacy's natural constituency of detractors will need something else to complain about.

February 1998

I loved being a food critic in the nineties. There was such a heady mix of wonderful and terrible cooking, both of which were often driven by the perceived need to be progressive, in flagrant, unashamed pursuit of the next big thing. So sometimes it was a pleasure and a relief to fall back on the kind of restaurant cooking that is quite simply impervious to the vagaries of fashion. And even if it wasn't that good, it still might be just what you wanted . . .

It's all Greek to me

It's not often I feel like a mediocre meal of burnt meat served with a so-so salad and a really filthy bottle of wine. But when I do, I always go to a Greek restaurant. And I am rarely disappointed.

The resolute refusal of the city high street Greek restaurants (invariably called the Aphrodite – or Apollo, or Acropolis – Taverna) to raise the level of their cooking, in keeping with the general improvement in the restaurant business in the last 20 years, is part of their unique charm. Even though you can now get taramasalata and humus in every corner shop, and takeaway kebab franchises now outnumber fish and chip shops, a couple of times a year it's nice to visit one of those 'traditional' Greek eateries – where they actually have chairs – if only to remind you why it is you haven't wanted to go for six months.

I conducted one of my biannual experiments with Greek cuisine last week. Only this time, I decided to try somewhere where the food had actually been recommended – and not by the second cousin of the wife of the brother of the man who owned the restaurant.

The place is Nontas, on Camden High Street, a long-running stalwart among Greek tavernas, which even merits a mention in the *Good Food Guide*. Happily, nothing about the dimly lit interior of the restaurant, or the dishes listed on the large, rather tatty fold-open menu, suggests that your experience will be any better than average. Indeed the prices – few starters are over £2, and the most expensive main course is a rump steak at £5.85 – lead you to expect the worst. So when the food turns out to be quite a lot better than okay, it's so surprising it's almost an affront.

The wine is equally noteworthy. When I tasted our bottle of well-chilled retsina, and said to the waiter 'Mmmm. This really is filthy,' he noted the tone of appreciation in my voice and said, with a sincere smile, 'Glad you like it.' He knew, of course, that a 'good bottle of retsina' is a contradiction in terms, and that the pleasure is all in the pain.

He really was an excellent waiter, responding to our pathetic indecision over the menu by steering us clear of dishes that he personally regarded as a little suspect: 'The *gemista* [marrow and vine leaves stuffed with rice and minced meat] really are much nicer than the *afelia* [pork cubes cooked in wine and coriander, served with *pourgouri*]. Trust me.'

We trusted, and were duly rewarded. After our standard Greek salads (no disappointment) the *gemista* was a winner (or should that be 'were winners'?), and so were the *keftedes* – pleasantly herby meatballs with a warm haricot bean salad. We also greedily ordered a single char-grilled quail, generously priced at £2.65 a bird. You couldn't say that it was rare, or even succulent. But there was much pleasure in its charred remains – the restaurant has a charcoal grill which produces that uniquely Greek style of burntness. Perhaps they throw some clever herbs over the hot coals.

We didn't test the puddings (although we did argue about the spelling of *paclava* – surely an initial 'b' is an option?). Instead we had Greek coffee (so called to distinguish it from Turkish coffee, which is exactly the same). Both were excellent: as good, in fact, as they are in Turkey.

So good was it all, that in an attempt to redress the balance of expectations, I took a step I would not normally contemplate, even when on holiday in Greece. I ordered a Metaxa brandy. This was really filthy, and ended the evening on the best possible note.

November 1991

The concept (did I use that word?) of the star chef began in the eighties. And in the nineties, the notion (that's better) became, like some of those thus described, a little tyrannical. It begged to be challenged . . .

Well done indeed!

Dining out at La Tante Claire seemed an excellent way to celebrate the publication of the 1993 edition of the *Good Food Guide*. No restaurant in the Guide receives higher praise. No chef has a greater reputation for accuracy and perfection than proprietor Pierre Koffman.

It also seemed as good a place as any to test a couple of editorial maxims in the new Guide that have received a certain amount of media attention: 'if a customer asks for his or her meat well done, chef has to do it' says the new Guide on page 659. To turn down a request for a second starter, in lieu of a main course, is, according to Guide editor Tom Jaine, 'wholly unreasonable.' How would the Guide's highest rated restaurant fare on these points of contention?

Two starters happened to be exactly what my dinner-mate wanted, and she was therefore able to order them without acting. 'Of course,' said our unblinking waiter (or was it 'no problem'? – I forget). For my main course I ordered the tornedos Rossini (fillet steak). 'I'd like that well done, please,' I said, my heart fluttering as I met the waiter's eye. 'Certainly sir,' he replied, without a hint of disapproval. 'Very well done, in fact,' I added for good measure. Did I detect a flicker of the eyebrow? I think I imagined it.

I had been put so utterly at my ease while making this philistine request that it was tempting to resummon the waiter. 'Only joking,' I wanted to say, 'Make mine a medium-rare.' But the mission would have been incomplete. What exactly would Koffman do to my steak?

My companion's second first course and my steak arrived. A more perfect interpretation of 'very well done' I could not conceive of. There was no question of bloodiness – little, in fact, of moisture. There were black crispy charred bits on the outside edges – which I imagine are relished by the aficionado of well done steaks. But charred though it was, you could not say any attempt had been made to sabotage the dish, and thereby teach me a lesson. This very well done-ness of this steak was – for want of a better phrase – very well done.

If there was a statement on my plate it was made by the slabs of foie gras with which this classic steak dish was generously garnished. Two fat pieces rested atop my frazzled filet. Tender, moist, and delicious, they were as good as foie gras can be – and perfectly pink in the middle. But then I hadn't asked for them any other way.

So if the mighty Koffman will do you a well done steak, who are the guilty culprits who will send you packing if you dare to raise the subject? Michel Perraud, formerly of Les Alouettes in Claygate, Surrey, is chastised in the new Guide for refusing to serve duck, venison, pigeon or lamb because a customer asked for them well done. The *Daily Mail* last week cited the ever-controversial Marco Pierre White, of Harvey's in Wandsworth, as another example of a chef who 'would not serve a well done steak'. I called him.

'Not true,' says White. 'Jaine came to my restaurant over three and a half years ago with some bimbo. She ordered a fore-rib of beef which she asked to be well done. We simply advised that that was not the best way to eat that particular cut – it would have been unpalatably tough. If they'd insisted, I would have done it, but they didn't. They ordered something else. Jaine has accused me of being a dictator to my customers ever since. Let's face it, the man's a c**t – and you can quote me on that. He's the scruffiest punter I've ever had in here.'

White went on to make this pledge: 'If you come to my restaurant and order nothing but a plate of vegetables, I'll give them to you. They'll be the most expensive vegetables in London, but I'll do them. And if you ask for a well done tornedos, I'll cut it into three, so I can cook it through without drying it out completely.'

Jaine himself denies that his comments were directed particularly at White, though he does say the *Mail* story was 'quite accurate, though it all happened a while ago'. The subject of White certainly raises his defences: 'I have no comment to make on that man.' When I suggested that Harvey's might be a good place to meet for lunch to discuss the problems of being a Guide editor, Jaine was unequivocal: 'Don't start mixing it, now.'

Though he refused to name any other red meat dictators ('I've been getting into trouble over this all day') Jaine was clear as to just what is bugging him on the restaurant scene: 'There is a large number of chefs who seem to think that the object of the game is to express their personality, whereas in fact the object of a restaurant is to feed hungry people.'

It's certainly a brave stand, but one that is ultimately undermined by the style of the *Good Food Guide* itself. The text is increasingly inclined to make distinctions between chefs on the finest points of expertise, and pronounce authoritatively on all elements of culinary style. That's why the punters, myself included, love to read it. But such a text is hardly a discouragement of the cult of the celebrity chef – witness also the number of entries that mention the chef by name, not just the information at the end, but throughout the text.

The thorny question is this: how can the Guide continue to celebrate the burgeoning talents of our most gifted chefs, whilst championing the consumer's right to eat burnt meat? Perhaps I could make a suggestion. I notice in this year's Guide two new symbols that appear prominently at the top of entries. A crossed-out cigarette butt indicates that a restaurant has a no smoking dining room; a £ sign suggests you can eat here for less than £20 a head, all in. Next year Mr Jaine might like to consider an addition to this useful shorthand: a charred fillet, with rising smoke. Restaurants marked by this sign will do your steak any way you like. Pierre Koffman would no doubt sport this symbol with pride.

October 1993

Understanding Marco

Marco Pierre White's large and slickly designed new menu – the cover is a Bob Carlos Clarke enlarged sepia-tint photograph of a pile of garlic cloves – has by way of a preface the following quote from Oscar Wilde: 'To get into society nowadays, one has to either feed people, amuse people, or shock people.' The implication seems to be that if, like White, you can manage all three, you will be well away.

And so, apparently, he is, for a visit to Harvey's is *de rigueur* for any major celebrity passing through London – despite being, as far as the metropolitan buzz is concerned – practically out in the sticks (Wandsworth).

The lunchtime I visited Harvey's, in the hope of being fed, amused and shocked by the notorious chef-patron, Ivana Trump had dined there the night before. According to White 'she ate like a horse' – and was so impressed that she asked him to provide the nosebags for a private function the following night. 'I don't usually do outside catering,' he explained, 'but the money she was offering – I couldn't refuse.' He went on to explain that he was a bit strapped for cash at the moment – 'had a very bad tip on the horses from a friend. Or rather an ex-friend.'

White had agreed to give me an interview and came to join my co-luncher and me at the tail end of our main course. 'I see you're having the *osso bucco*,' he said, dipping his finger several times in rapid succession into the rich, ginger-spiked sauce on my plate and then into his mouth. 'This sauce isn't quite right yet – should be a bit thicker.' He then picked up a fork from the (unoccupied) next door table, and we duelled over the remaining meat on the shin bone. I'd like to think I won the battle for the bone marrow, but it was close.

He ordered our puddings for us – raspberry millefeuille for my lunchmate and the stunning apricot soufflé–omelette for me. I wasn't taking any chances and rapidly wolfed down my omelette, losing out only on a couple of apricot halves which White speared with his index finger. My companion was not so lucky – her mistake was to show some indecision over her millefeuille. Without a word of warning our host picked it up, broke it in half, and shoved the larger portion in his mouth like a greedy child with an illicit cream slice. 'That's how you should eat my millefeuille,' he said, picking up the remaining half and propelling it with alarming speed towards my mouth. 'Now it's your turn . . . Well done!' It was completely delicious – but the bit of Marco's finger that came with it wasn't quite such a thrill.

By now the tablecloth was richly decorated with cream and crushed raspberries, and White had given a new meaning to the phrase '*le patron mange ici*'. I gave up trying to tackle the exuberant chef with my list of questions. Instead we listened to him hold forth on his three favourite subjects: food, fishing and sex. I wouldn't like to commit myself as to which of these is his foremost passion. On this occasion all three were given a good airing: 'You should have had the sea bass caviar,' (his new signature dish which has a £25 supplement on the set menu) '. . . it's just fantastic! . . . have you seen the new Shimano baitrunner reels – they're unbelievable . . . I wonder where I could get a pair of medieval stocks . . .'

In fairness to White, his most exuberant antics are generally reserved for journalists, whom he no doubt considers fair game, and friends, whom he knows can take it. At the same lunch he was charm itself to another table of bona fide diners, who were clearly delighted, if initially a little nervous, to meet the *enfant terrible*. Nevertheless, something about his wild-eyed manner and pent-up energy made me realise that White's occasional outbursts and boisterous behaviour are not mere stunts of showmanship or publicity seeking. They are intrinsic parts of his complex character. The blessing is that somehow, in the kitchen, the energy and the anarchy are trammelled into a controlled creative process that allows him to produce imaginative but intense dishes of unqualified and consistent excellence. The aforementioned *osso bucco* is a case in point. His own criticism of the sauce shows his extraordinary level of perfectionism, finding fault with a dish that we thought could not have been improved upon.

White's latest venture is a new restaurant in Chelsea Harbour. Harvey's Canteen, a joint project with Langan's Brasserie proprietor Michael Caine, will seat 150 and serve a simplified brasserie version of White's distinctive cuisine. It opens in September. 'I'm hoping that many more beautiful women will come and eat at the Canteen than I can currently fit into Harvey's,' was all he would reveal about it. I wouldn't bet against it.

June 1993

Ego, often displayed as sky-high confidence, may not be an essential ingredient of culinary stardom – but it certainly seems to help. When I first met Jean-Christophe Novelli, his confidence seemed to make fame and fortune almost inevitable.

Modest – moi?

'See you on Monday night, then,' said the heavily accented French voice on the telephone. 'And by the way – I think you will be impressed.'

The owner of the voice is Jean-Christophe Novelli, chef-patron of a restaurant called Provence at Gordleton Mill, a small country house hotel on the edge of the New Forest. Novelli is perhaps not yet a name on the lips of every foodie, but he is tipped by many to become a big star on the English restaurant scene.

His parting remark on the telephone smacked of arrogance – but let's not be too English. I have always had a sneaking admiration for the Gallic lack of modesty. I remember my cousin's French exchange, a girl of only 15, but of a physique and aloof beauty way out of my league. The only chat-up lines I could muster were things like 'Do you play tennis?' and 'Do you like swimming?' The answer was always, 'Yes, and I am very good.' She turned out to be right in every case. It made me long to ask about some other things I thought she might be good at, but of course I never dared.

As we sat in the charming garden by the millstream, we had our first chance to find out if Novelli's confidence – in the kitchen department, that is – was equally justified. With our pre-dinner drinks we were served a piece of cucumber, cleverly sculpted into the shape of a crab. Two large opalescent salmon eggs, each topped with a tiny black bead of caviar, were the crab's goggling eyes. So now we know Novelli can carve vegetables, but can he cook?

God, yes. The tone was set by the appetiser – a single fat scallop served in its shell on a bed of noodles, topped with a julienne of cucumber, the whole dressed with the lightest of butter sauces. It was a treat of slippery textures and succulent shellfish.

Novelli does not shrink from crediting his mentors – he later explained that this dish was adapted from a recipe devised by his friend Marco Pierre White, who does something similar with oysters. But the next course was all his own. He calls it a *barigoule froide simple au blanc de tourteaux et anchoïade,* although how the word '*simple*' gets in I'm not quite sure. The English translation on the menu tells you all you need to know: 'Braised artichoke infused with olive oil and lime, filled with fresh, white crab meat and diced avocado, flavoured with anchovy mayonnaise, encased in thick slices of home-smoked salmon and topped with a gently poached quail's egg and caviar.'

Original combinations and complex techniques feature strongly on the menu and, in the dishes we sampled, were handled with a panache tempered by precision. Roast lamb cutlets were filled with a light Stilton mousse and served on a fricassee of lentils, and scallops reappeared (well, we ordered them) layered between sheets of filo pastry, flavoured with lemon grass, with asparagus and pistachio.

Desserts are Novelli's finest hour. This year he won the Häagen-Dazs award for Dessert of the Year with a Fabergé-like nougatine box filled with chocolate mousse and with caramel springs bursting out the top. We chose a less elaborate crème brûlée, classic but for a subtle flavouring of coconut, and a peach tarte tatin, perhaps the best version of that pudding, with its sticky, caramelised pastry, that I have ever eaten.

Novelli greeted us at the end of our meal with the twinkling eye of an actor who knows very well that he has held an audience in the palm of his hand. Indeed he went on to say that he considered cooking to be a performance art. 'Here we do two shows, lunch and dinner, and each one we try to make better than the last. My team is like a group of actors. We have to work well together, and hopefully we can produce something a bit special.'

It's a very young group. Novelli has just turned 30, his deputy chef is 19, and his restaurant manager, who handles the front of the house with confidence and charm, is just 20.

I hope they will stay together. Novelli has a reputation as something of a rolling stone, rarely staying in a restaurant kitchen for more than a year.

'I was impatient,' he admits, 'but only because I was in a hurry to be in a place where I can cook food exactly how I want it to be. I have always wanted to be a chef-manager – to be in charge of a place, to be independent and run a place entirely in my way. I have that here – and I will stay.' And as long as he does, culinary enthusiasts who find themselves in the south of England will have a vital port of call.

Go and see for yourself. And by the way – I think that you'll be impressed.

April 1993

When chefs accrue the status of gastro-gods, then the foodie fans who worship at their temples – aka restaurants – can also get a little extreme. And, like all extremists, they will inevitably form gangs and argue.

Perfection – purely academic

'This wine is like a ballerina, who dances quite beautifully, but never smiles,' said the gastronome opposite me, with a sigh. 'Spirits, you see, mature on a logarithmic rather than a linear scale, so the key-tones take a long time to develop,' said the gastronome on my left, drawing a graph in the air with his glass.

Gastronomy is defined as the art or science of good eating and drinking. Gastronomes, correspondingly, seem to divide neatly in their approach to their sacred subject, into artists and scientists. For some, food is sheer pleasure, every meal a new adventure. For others, it is the relentless pursuit of perfection. I didn't say that, by the way. It was another gastronome.

I heard such pearls as a guest of the British Academy of Gastronomes at their monthly dinner, last Tuesday. On this occasion, the dinner was at the Dorchester. This was in itself an excitement for the Academy, as the Dorchester restaurant has been closed for refurbishment for almost two years. Previously, under the control of that big Swiss cheese Anton Mosimann, it achieved the dizzy heights of Michelin two-stardom. The new chef, Willi Elsener, is also Swiss and was formerly Mosimann's *second de cuisine*. But, according to the strict rules of the Michelin Guide, he must start from scratch.

Elsener's menu was presented, as is traditional at these dinners, by one of the gastronomes, on this occasion Egon Ronay, a founder member of the Academy. He had collaborated with the chef over the previous fortnight, and come up with a menu to excite and challenge the palates of his fellow experts.

While the delights to come were lovingly described by Mr Ronay, I took stock of those experts. The Academy are, in fact, a band of happy amateurs. Most members have no connection with the food business, but are lawyers, bankers, publishers, industrialists, writers. And, unlike the French Academy (on which it is modelled), some are women. The membership list boasts a few well-known names – Len Deighton, Sandy Gall, Patrick Lichfield – but their celebrity is incidental to what binds them together, that they care, and know, a very great deal about food.

Our *amuse-gueules*, which were not described by Mr Ronay on our menus, were little deep-fried balls of batter, with something green inside. 'What's this?' said one gastronome, clearly stumped. 'It could be a slither of courgette, or even cucumber,' ventured another.

I was able to play my trump card at this point. 'It tastes like a sage leaf to me,' I said, quietly. 'What's that you say? Sage? Yes, I do believe you're right.' A murmur of assent spread around the table. A few suspicious looks came my way, too. These were entirely justified, as my 'lucky guess' was in fact a sure thing. A prior consultation with the menu-proposer has its advantages.

It was my turn to be amazed when the next course arrived, first at the sheer beauty of the thing, and then at the experts' assessment of it. It was a mousse of lobster, in shocking pink, filled with little pieces of lobster meat flavoured *à l'Americaine*, and served on a bed of winter leaves.

After some generally appreciative noises, the real analysis began: 'The flavour is good, but could be stronger.' 'The filling is better than the mousse, which is too firm.' 'The salad leaves are underdressed, and anyway the dressing needs more acidity. Some citrus perhaps.' These gastronomes took no prisoners.

The next course was a simple chicken consommé, clear as crystal and the colour of fine pale brandy. In it floated a single raviolo, filled with a light stuffing of vegetables, minced chicken, and a hint of tomato. The purity of this concept seemed to strike a chord with the assembly. It was hailed as a masterpice: 'So clean and clear.' 'Quite beautiful.' 'The best chicken consommé I have ever had.'

There was high praise, too, for the venison, served with an earthy combination of mushrooms (as a topping), puréed Brussels sprouts with chestnuts, tiny crisp potatoes and a sauce of fresh cranberries. It was robust, accessible, and quite delicious.

'Very artisanal. Almost peasanty,' said my neighbour. 'As is the Côtes-du-Rhône,' said his.

Dessert was a sorbet, the most delicate of rose whites, made from pink champagne. It arrived in an almond tuile basket, garnished with exotic fruits. The sorbet was exquisite; but a coating of dark chocolate at the base of the tuile was generally agreed to detract from the subtlety of the fruits. Its presence was functional. It served as a waterproofing for the tuile, so that the juices from the fruits would not make it soggy.

At the end of the Academy meal, the proposer is answered by an assessor. In this case, the role was undertaken by a former inspector for Egon Ronay's guide, the shipping broker Aristodimos Sofianos. In the true gastronomic spirit, he pulled no punches. Though he found much to praise, especially the consommé and venison, he was candid about the mousse: 'Something was missing here. It was too bland.'

After the assessment, the chairman of the Dorchester board of directors, Lord Bramall, was heard to mutter to himself: 'We must not be too bland.' It seemed a good thought to take home.

December 1990

Away from the dazzling world of star chefs and their high concept eateries, 'normal' food life — breakfast, elevenses, lunch, tea, supper — is still what sustains most of us, most of the time. But even breakfast cereals and biscuits are not impervious to the vagaries of hype and fashion . . .

Snap, crackles and hype

I would like to begin this week by casting my vote in the great 'Golden' debate currently raging amongst those who rightly believe breakfast to be the most important meal of the day. The Grahams have it; the Crackles are, frankly, not even close.

I am, of course, talking about breakfast cereal. Two of the most hyped breakfast cereals, in fact, since Kellogg's launched Crunchy Nut Cornflakes with a massive fanfare some six years ago, and enriched the lives of brekophiles everywhere. You had to hand it to Kellogg's for that; they really cleaned up with CNCs. Now, however, they have missed their mark, both with their advertising, and their product. The TV ad ludicrously attempts to imply that anyone who does not eat Golden Crackles (who are fighting for Kellogg's in the cereal war) will get rained on, whereas those who do will enjoy a lifelong blessing of golden sunshine.

I ate my first bowl of Crackles a few weeks ago one Sunday morning in the garden. Sometime around my third or fourth mouthful, it began to drizzle. This hardly mattered, as my first mouthful had already shown me that this product was going to bring no metaphorical sunshine to my taste buds, even if it could bring perennial Hawaiian rays. They also have that defect common to several recently launched Kellogg's cereals. Like the now discontinued Start (which faded simultaneously with the man who swore by them, Steve Cram), and the let's-hope-soon-to-be-discontinued Honey Nut Loops (far too sweet), Crackles will lacerate your mouth to shreds if you do not let them soak in the milk for a good while. And if you do let them soak, well then naturally they'll be all soggy and horrid. So You Just Can't Win With Crackles. And perhaps I might suggest that as the strapline in all their future advertising.

Meanwhile Nestlé's Golden Grahams have completely won me

over. It was, admittedly, an amazing piece of luck that their complimentary miniature promotional box happened to land on my doormat only seconds after I had discovered that my flatmate's all-guzzling younger brother had pilfered the last of the CNCs, and that there was nothing in the fridge but a scant quarter pint of milk. But What Really Got Me Was The Taste (and there's another one for the red glasses brigade). Described on the packet as 'crispy golden squares of corn and wholewheat, coated in honey and brown sugar', they are somewhere between a Shreddie and a Crunchy Nut Cornflake – which I'm sure you'll agree is a pretty exciting place to be. They are indeed crispy, without being abrasive, and the coating is so cleverly applied that they retain their crispness in milk quite long enough for one to finish a bowl before encountering the sensation that one is eating finely chopped wet newspaper.

Their ad campaign gets a thumbs up too. Instead of claiming to control the weather, or featuring shameless prats with impeded speech and a Hawaiian shirt singing badly scanning couplets about 'eating it by the case', they patiently try to explain to bemused potential customers how such a magnificent breakfast cereal got landed with such an idiotic name. (And let's face it, even when applied to animate objects Graham is a very silly name.) I can't remember off hand what the explanation was, but I remember finding it very convincing, and being pleased that it had nothing whatever to do with any individual called Graham.

August 1991

Dunk food takes the biscuit

Hail Dunkers is a new biscuit on the supermarket shelves, specially made for those who like to dip something crisp and dry into something hot and wet, and suck on the resulting gunge.

If that sounds crude, then I make no apology. Dunking is crude. At least it is regarded as crude by a hefty minority of the population. According to a Mori poll taken earlier this year, 52 per cent of us think that it's 'all right to dunk', while 38 per cent regard the habit as 'socially unacceptable'.

The young (15- to 35-year-olds), it transpires, are more inclined to dunk than the old, with the over-55s branded 'least likely to dunk'. This comes as no great surprise, when you consider the prevalence of dentures among the upper age bracket. Dunking is not denture-friendly.

The geographical epidemiology of dunking was also considered. The survey revealed that the concentration of people who will not stoop to dunk is particularly high (54 per cent) among the genteel Scots (who are also inclined to hold their saucer in one hand, their cup in the other, and cock their little finger when they sip their tea – a body language which leaves no hands or digits free for dunking).

Like so many polls, this one sadly leaves the really interesting questions unanswered. For a start, the survey is only concerned with whether or not people dunk.

This assumes that all dunkers are the same – which is, of course, nonsense. For a start, dunkers must choose their biscuits. There are those who dunk only one sort, and those who are promiscuous. Other variables include time, depth and frequency of immersion.

Number-crunchers like me want some harder facts about the wet biscuit-munchers. This is my suggested list of questions for the next major poll on Britain's dunking habits:

1) What biscuits do you regularly dunk?

2) What biscuits would you never dunk?

3) How much of the biscuit is dipped in the drink?

4) How long do you leave it there?

5) Do you dunk before every bite, or do you intersperse drinking with dry biting?

6) Do you eat the soggy crumbs left at the bottom of your cup?

7) If the soggy end falls off, do you scoop it out with a teaspoon and eat it straightaway?

Such imponderables aside, we must consider the future of the newcomer to the biscuit shelf, Prewett Food's designer Dunker.

With so many exponents of this activity at large in the UK, a biscuit specifically designed (ovoid, no less) for dunking, sounds, on the face of it, like a cunning marketing wheeze. I have my doubts.

My own theory – which I have no intention of asking Mori to investigate by poll – is that regular dunkers (I don't mean the new biscuit, I mean those who dunk) are by nature very conservative people. The act of dunking – rendering sloppy and amorphous, and eventually disintegrating – a biscuit that was, only moments before, crisp, pristine and complete, is about the most rebellious thing that most of them ever do. To dunk, for them, is to commit an act of anarchy.

Such defiant gestures are not undertaken lightly; in particular, they are not undertaken with unfamiliar biscuits. Dunkers have their favourite biscuits, and they are not likely to switch overnight to some new-fangled, Johnny-come-lately brand.

The only way in which Dunkers (and now I am talking about the biscuit) can succeed is if they prove to be so far superior, when hot, wet and soggy, to other biscuits, that a single trial will convert even the most die-hard dunker of Digestives, or the most avid Ginger Nut nutter.

With this faint possibility in mind, I have conducted a comparative dunking of the new pretender with five household-name biscuit brands known to be among the nation's favourites for dunking.

The points of comparison are those I consider to be most salient to dunkers everywhere (even if they've never actually thought about it). They are: the speed with which the liquid is absorbed (some knowledge of this is essential for good timing of your dunk); the pleasantness (or otherwise) of the consistency of the totally saturated biscuit; and the advisability of dunking the biscuit in coffee as an occasional alternative to tea (which is, of course, the primary dunking beverage).

To dip or not to dip? And for how long? The good dunker's guide to the perfect coffee break

SOA = Speed Of Absorption
CWS = Consistency When Soggy
CWC = Compatibility With Coffee

Dunkers (Prewett's)

SOA: Fast
CWS: Retains some crunch, which is sugary rather than biscuity. Never goes completely soggy, even after three minutes' immersion.
CWC: Good. Unsweetened coffee helps to counteract the biscuit's excessive sweetness.
Verdict: Good for a couple of dunks, but ultimately too sweet. Dunkers who like their biscuits to become completely soggy are likely to be disappointed.
6/10

Rich Tea (McVities)

SOA: Medium slow
CWS: Totally soggy – smooth and creamy, melts in the mouth.
CWC: Takes on plenty of coffee flavour, as its own taste is mild and bland.
Verdict: A fine dunker. With good timing (about five seconds' immersion), it can be eaten when slippery and wet on the outside and still a tiny bit crunchy in the middle. Which is nice.
7/10

Digestives (McVities)

SOA: Medium fast
CWS: Soggy, but retains some granular texture (the nutty bran from the wholemeal flour can still be caught between the teeth).
CWC: Good, if you don't mind the saltiness (see below).
Verdict: A classic for dunking which is above criticism. The Digestive is saltier than most other sweet biscuits, which I have a problem with. Millions don't.
8/10

Garibaldi (Crawford's)

SOA: Fast
CWS: Totally soggy and wet, but for the middle layer of jammy, water-resistant currants.

CWC: Currants and coffee are not a great combo – best stick with tea.
Verdict: An acquired taste – for speciality dunkers only.
4/10

Ginger Nuts (McVities)

SOA: Medium slow
CWS: A pleasant granular texture even when completely soggy.
CWC: Excellent, and the basis, in fact, of a rather fine pudding: ginger biscuits soaked in strong coffee and sandwiched together with whipped cream.
Verdict: A truly great biscuit, whether dunked or not. Particularly good after a very short (three second) dunk, when they are wet but still crunchy.
9/10

Bourbon Creams (Crawford's)

SOA: Fast
CWS: Dunk an inch for more than ten seconds and it is guaranteed to fall off when you bring it back to the horizontal.
CWC: The chocolate combines with coffee for a delightful mocha effect.
Verdict: The creamy bit in the middle adds a whole new dimension; it melts, thereby allowing a deeply satisfying technique of combined dunking and licking.
7/10

August 1993

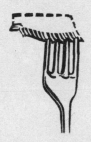

Home on the Range

**After all, food is first
and foremost a
family affair**

All the following pieces describe, in the loosest possible sense, my 'domestic' life with food, from my own childhood memories, to the daily business (and pleasure!) of feeding my own young family here at home. It seems to make sense to put them roughly in chronological order – of the recalled and recounted experiences, that is, not the writing.

Playing with food

'What can I do, Mum, I'm bored!' was a phrase heard often in our house when I was growing up – especially when it was raining outside – and I was invariably the one uttering it. Mum, who was probably trying to get some drawing done for her studies as a landscape gardener, had an infuriating way of answering this question – patiently, without looking up from her work, and with a generous smile:

'Well you could read a book . . . or paint a picture . . . or do a jigsaw . . . or play with your Lego, or . . .' the list of perfectly reasonable suggestions seemed practically endless, and as I knew she was teasing me I would be wincing and groaning and scuffing the carpet, saying 'bor-ing, bor-ing, bor-ing . . .'

She knew what I wanted to hear, and if she didn't say it soon enough, I would have to say it for her; '. . . make peppermint creams?' I'd enquire, with a hopeless attempt at nonchalance, as if I was merely trying to help her in her quest for a sensible suggestion. 'Well, I suppose you could . . .'

My sister Sophy and I both loved cooking with Mum – when she was doing pastry, we'd get to make jam tarts with the trimmings. When she went through a bread-making phase, we'd be allowed to customise our own little loaves: my sister would plait three strands of dough together very neatly, while I would shove as many raisins as I was allowed to get away with into my lumpy bread rolls.

But after she went back to college Mum had less time for cooking, and less time to indulge us with her constant presence. Sophy was as good at entertaining herself as I was hopeless. She would read voraciously, fill whole books with her drawings and invent frighteningly complex versions of solitaire using a chess set. I would hang around Mum's drawing board doing everything I could to induce parental guilt. I couldn't believe her resistance.

Making peppermint creams was the magic solution to this stand-off. It was the first bit of cooking at which I was allowed to go solo. There were (and still are) just four ingredients: icing sugar, egg white, peppermint essence and green colouring. And, most importantly, no cooking is required, so there was no need for me to go anywhere near the cooker.

To begin with, Mum would have to set me up for the session. Weigh out the icing sugar into a bowl. Separate the egg. Dust the rolling pin with icing sugar. Scatter some more across the table for rolling out on (in a beautiful even layer that was a wonder to behold). She'd probably get ten minutes' respite before she'd be summoned back into the kitchen with an agonised, tear-surpressing cry: 'Mum . . . Mum . . . it's all gone wrong.' I'd have iced my hands, my face, the table and the rolling pin in minty green goo. She'd scrape me down, reassemble the sugar dough to perfect rolling consistency, and help me roll it out . . .

She'd probably get another five minutes' work in while I made a start at stamping out rounds with a little pastry cutter. Then it would be, 'Mum . . . Mum . . . help . . . they're all sticking to the table!' Any incentive to improve my technique was minimal. I realised, not quite consciously perhaps, that if I made enough of a hash of things, I could usually get Mum to abandon her work, and stay with me until the session was finished, and the cool green patties were laid out on a tray in neat rows. Then I would get to lick the bowl and the spoon, while she did the washing up.

Nonetheless, I made peppermint creams so often that in the end I couldn't help but get good at it. Really good at it. Soon I could knock off a set in about 20 minutes flat, including the cleaning up. Then I would be back in my mother's office, destroying the carpet.

So I graduated to chocolate-dipped peppermint creams – so elegant that Mum would serve them with pride (mine and hers) with the coffee at the end of her dinner parties. To make these required heat – enough to melt a couple of bars of Meunier chocolate (I was in love with the yellow-green wrappers). But Mum could double up the stove work with a coffee break from her studies, boiling the kettle, then placing the Pyrex bowl of broken chocolate squares over a pan of just boiled water. She could then go back to work with her coffee, while I was entrusted to stir the bowl above the pan until the chocolate was smooth and flowing.

When I was finished with dipping, or half-dipping, the peppermint creams, there was usually a significant pool of chocolate left in the bottom of the bowl. Often more than I could realistically manage on my own, as chef's perks. So I would try and improvise some gleeful tea-time treat, stirring in a little butter, golden syrup or honey, along with handfuls of raisins, Cornflakes or Rice Crispies, or maybe broken Digestive biscuits.

Squished into a tray, these concoctions might or might not set firm when placed in the fridge. If they did, they could be cut into squares, and served up for tea. If they didn't, we'd attack the goo in the tray, with spoons. Mum, Soph and I could easily clear a batch in a single sitting.

In the end, the only way Mum could hope to get any peace was to buy me a pair of oven gloves and begin to train me up on the safe use of the cooker. Inevitably cakes, biscuits, eclairs and profiteroles soon began to flow from my endeavours. By the age of ten I was boiling up fudge, toffee and Turkish delight with, it seemed to me, only the merest hint of adult supervision.

By now I was equipped with the best weapons against boredom that any boy could wish for: a sugar thermometer, a piping bag, and a well-stocked store cupboard. And, most importantly, an infinitely kind, loving and patient Mum.

June 2005

Hooked by a tricky fish

When I was five years old my father took me fishing for the first time, in Richmond Park. The water in question was a tiny stream, barely a trickle, and the tackle somewhat primitive: a bamboo cane with a length of string and a safety pin tied to the end. Despite my tender years, and total ignorance of the subtle art of the angle, I had a pretty good idea that Dad's tactics, and choice of fishing ground, left a bit to be desired.

After about 30 seconds of patiently holding the rod, boredom began to set in. Dad suggested that I should take a stroll down the bank – which may sound irresponsible, but an inch-and-a-half of water doesn't pose much of a threat to a buoyant, porky five-year-old – and if any excitement should occur, he would summon me with a yell.

Amazingly, I had hardly wandered more than about 15 yards away when well-rehearsed shouts of 'Come quick, I think we've got this one!' had me running back to his side. He handed me the rod and in a state of high excitement I hauled a good size fish on to the bank. Before I had time to satisfy my considerable curiosity over this previously unstudied form of life, my father had grasped it firmly around the middle and smacked it three times on the head with a large stick. 'Mustn't let it escape,' he explained, and then presented a very dead fish for my examination. I was most impressed by the swiftness of this dispatch, and could only conclude that my father knew more about the ways of the river than I had previously supposed. And as far as the sport of fishing was concerned, I was hooked.

Back at home I got busy with my *Observer's Book of Fishes* and identified our catch as a mackerel. Nor did I fail to notice that, according to my reference book, the mackerel is a fish that lives in the sea. When I pointed this out to my other prime source of information, the omniscient Dad, he had, of course, an entirely convincing explanation: 'It must have decided to swim up from the sea, like salmon do.'

Meanwhile my mother fried our catch in butter, and served it to me with a wedge of lemon. I wasn't allowed ketchup either. And so, probably for the first time, I devoured and thoroughly enjoyed a piece of fish that was neither finger-shaped, nor covered in orange breadcrumbs.

It was ten years before the truth of that day's events came out. Something about the sight of his 15-year-old son swearing blind to his disbelieving friends that he had caught a mackerel in a Richmond Park ditch with a pellet of Mother's Pride on a safety pin finally moved my father to make a confession – about the trip to the fishmonger's, the subtle ploy of sending me off for a walk, the quick dispatch lest I should discover that my catch was already quite dead.

I was disillusioned, even angry for a while. But ultimately I was grateful. For I had learned some important lessons, that could not be unlearned merely by the revelation that I had been the victim of a deceit. I had learned, for example, always to expect the unexpected when fishing; never to underestimate the potential of an unexplored piece of water to produce a catch; and, most important of all, I had discovered the unmatched joy of cooking and eating a self-caught fish. And I relish it to this day.

January 1993

And that's just for starters

I remember my first real restaurant experience as clearly as my first two-wheeled bicycle (a Raleigh Chipper, if you were wondering). I was six years old when my parents were invited by friends to have lunch one summer Sunday at the The Hole in the Wall, in Bath. Since it said in the 1971 *Good Food Guide*, 'children welcome', it was decided that my sister and I could go too.

To start with I had smoked salmon and brown bread, which made such a deep impression on me that for the next five years at least, whenever anyone asked me what my favourite food was, I said 'smokedsalmonandbrownbread' without hesitation. I chose the Sunday roast for my main course, and it arrived on a trolley under a silver dome big enough to hide in. My dad tells me he's never seen my eyes bulging with such anticipation before or since. The waiter said, 'You can have as much as you like', a phrase which resonates deeply in the mind, and stomach, of a six-year-old.

Pudding was strawberries: a huge glass bowl of them came with another invitation to indulge without limit. So when I couldn't eat any more, I put the biggest one I could find in the middle of my heavy linen napkin, and squashed it on the table with my fist. As I watched the crimson juices spread slowly up the napkin, I felt about as drunk on the whole scene as my parents were on Pimms and Chianti.

It was a seminal experience – the moment I learned, though I wouldn't fully understand it for some years, that eating in a restaurant can be (even if it very rarely is) a uniquely stimulating passage of hours that creates a brief narrative in one's life of near-perfect structure: starter, main course, pudding. Simple but brilliant.

Now I am the parent and the boot is on the other foot. Of course I want Oscar (nearly four) to realise what a delight it can be to eat in restaurants. But I don't want to spoil him, and make him blasé, by over-exposing him to the culture before he's able to appreciate it. On the other hand, if we're going out to eat, and it suits us, for whatever reason, to take him with us, then why should we dumb down to pizza or burgers (unless that happens to be exactly what we fancy eating)? We'll go where we want to go, and provided we're all made to feel welcome, he'll come too.

The result is that Oscar has already eaten in dozens of restaurants, including some very good ones. His eating-out career began as a swathed and sleeping baby, continued as a restless and demanding toddler, and has blossomed these last few months as a valid, if somewhat junior punter, with a marked interest in the menu and strong sense of what items on it he does or doesn't fancy.

If you ask him which is his favourite restaurant, he will answer, 'Arthur's', referring to Arthur Watson, proprietor of The Riverside Restaurant in West Bay, Dorset, which, as well as being one of the finest fish restaurants in the southwest, is arguably the most child-friendly restaurant in the country. Why? Because they understand that the secret of being child-friendly is nothing more or less than being friendly to children – and specifically doesn't involve paper hats, dinosaur-shaped chicken pieces, and addressing the entire party as if they are all under-fives (as in 'have you been to a Harvester before?').

If you ask him what's the best thing he's ever had in a restaurant, he'll say, 'the little fish' and if you push for clarification by asking 'which little fish?' he might elaborate, 'the ones when I did a pee'. He's referring to a meal a few months back at Moro, in Exmouth Market, where we went *à deux* and ate fresh anchovies. They came chargrilled, with a dressing of fresh mint, thyme, garlic and lemon. The experience of munching them up, heads, tails and all, while licking this fishy, herby elixir off our fingers, was so exquisite and diverting that Oscar apparently decided that, on balance, wet pants were preferable to a troublesome trip to the loo.

And if you ask him which is the last restaurant he went to, he may or may not remember that it is called St John, even though we went there yesterday. But he'll tell you that the crispy pig's skin and watercress salad 'was nice, but it wasn't really fair, because it didn't say it would have capers', and that the chocolate cake with vanilla ice cream was 'the bestest, yummiest, scrummiest in my tummiest ever ever ever!'. And he must have forgiven the capers, because on the way out he asked, 'Daddy, can we come to this restaurant every time we're in London?'

So I wonder which, if any of these, will be his Hole in the Wall. Has he had his seminal restaurant moment already, or is it yet to come? With a bit of luck, one day, he'll tell me.

January 2003

When I left home for university, food came with me, and I took every opportunity to inflict my passion and my prejudices on my fellow students – not just in person, but in print.

This is my first ever published food article, written for the university magazine. There is a whiff of youthful over-exuberance about it, but I don't find it too embarrassing to re-read (compared to the one on page 156). The baked beans recipe is an old favourite adapted from one in a lovely kid's cookbook, called Cooking is a Game You Can Eat, *by Fay Maschler. I should have credited her at the time – but that's students for you. I still make it, once or twice a year, to this day.*

The two things that resonate most about the piece, though, are that the M&S avocado and prawn sandwich is hailed as the height of exotica, and Bulgarian wine is poised to become the essential lubricant of all student social activity. It all comes flooding back . . .

A hill of beans

It is well known (not to say palpably obvious) that Oxford students differ considerably as to race, creed, colour, political persuasion, sexual persuasion, interests, pastimes and hobbies. But there is one thing that they all think about approximately three times a day, and that is food. And the hobby that comes a close second (more popular even than hacking) is the consumption of alcoholic drink. So it is with great pleasure that I welcome you to the all-new food and drink page (or possibly column, by the time the editors have whipped out their carving knives and separated the fat and gristle from the lean meat).

It could be argued that a great number of Oxford students do not think about food at all. They merely subconsciously gravitate towards the nearest source of chips. As far as I am concerned, such types are, foodly speaking, philistines – beyond redemption (and the pale). But I am an optimist, and believe the chip-eaters to be a dwindling minority.

For those who have not sunk so low, but whose eating habits are stuck in the rut of fried breakfast and baked beans three times a day, here is a recipe:

Mean beanz

1 small (or half a large) onion; 1 large tin beans; 1 tsp mustard; 1 splurge ketchup; 1 tbsp Worcestershire sauce

Fry the onion (chop it up first) until brown. Then add the beans. Add the mustard, ketchup and Worcestershire sauce (not necessarily in that order). Then heat until hot. Do not boil or overheat as this impairs flavour (cf. back of baked bean tin). This is a Jekyll-to-Hyde transformation from boring, bland baked beans to a daring, witty accompaniment to the usual fried breakfast. Also delicious on toast. An even more flamboyant alternative replaces the Worcestershire sauce with a heaped teaspoon (mild) or two (hot) of curry powder and adds half an apple (chopped) plus about 40 raisins.

These recipes will serve two pigs or three gourmets. If not polluted with fried sausages, fried egg, fried bread and fried bacon, Mean beanz are actually very healthy, the beans being protein-packed and the onion and apple very vitaminous.

Before we move on to higher things (see next issue, 'Planning a Party') a brief word about the sandwich. Students are much given to eating sandwiches, and the good news is that, unlike the chip-eaters, sandwich-eaters are not held in complete contempt by civilised *mangeurs*. Eating sandwiches is ideologically quite sound. The major sandwich outlet in Oxford is the polythene-wrapped Breadline product, delivered fresh daily and sold in a number of newsagents and corner shops, most notably (or centrally) Wendy News and The Tuck Shop. Pretty good sarnies, these, available in both white and wholemeal, and fairly generously filled. The fillings are hardly imaginative, though, being variations on the traditional egg and cress, cheese and pickle, ham and salad themes.

More exotic, but also more expensive, are the Marks and Sparks product – including BLT, prawn cocktail, egg and bacon, and even avocado and prawn, as well as the more usual cheese and ham variations. The salady ones always have good crisp lettuce and plenty of mayo. There is a sandwich bar by the main entrance, so you don't have to queue up in the food department.

Those who like to take their sandwiches sitting down, and perhaps with a friend, should go to George's in the Covered Market. He will construct a sandwich to your specification. George's also do toasties, and to my mind the best sandwich available in Oxford is a George's hot bacon and mushroom number – a true butty, this: greedy, greasy, great.

Sandwich snobs will already be familiar with Hero's, where pitta bread is split and filled to make the trendiest, most upmarket sandwiches in town. Hero's is rightfully popular, but not cheap enough for a true butty-buff, and one is liable to queue there.

For a superb sandwich filling which will keep for days in the fridge, try mashing a 7oz tin of tuna with two hard-boiled eggs, half an onion (finely chopped), a small carton of yoghurt and a good blob of mayo. Season well with salt and pepper.

It has been pointed out to me that a review of the Oxford sandwich scene would not be complete without mentioning Don Miller's Hot Bread Kitchen (Queen Street). So I just did.

Best wine buys

Buy Bulgarian. That's the hot tip at the moment, for both red and white. Cabernet Sauvignon (1979 if you can find it, 1981 will do) at just over £2 a bottle is a red wine well worth drinking while you're still sober, unlike most reds at that price. And the white Pinot Chardonnay is blissfully free of the caustic afterburn that seems *de rigueur* for most cheap whites. A crisp, dry white, and it's a snip at around £1.90.

October 1986

I had a London infancy, a country boyhood, went to a town university and spent my twenties working in the capital and playing, as often as possible, in the country at weekends. By the end of my third decade of unresolved rural-urban dual identity, something had to give. River Cottage beckoned . . .

In the end, the move to Dorset hasn't just changed the way I live, but also the way I think, the things I believe are important, and therefore what I choose to write about. It is a pure coincidence, but a charming one I think, that the piece below, chronicling the slow journey towards what now seems inevitable, was published on Valentine's Day.

Taking the cure, instead of the car

Until this time last year, I was one of millions suffering from an increasingly common late-twentieth-century malaise. Those of us who have been afflicted know it is a suffocating condition, all the more so because the medical community refuses to acknowledge our pain and disorientation. It has been said we 'borrow' our symptoms from a range of known psycho-social traumas, including split personality, transvestism and compulsive-obsessive behaviour. Those who are diagnosed with these conditions get help. Yet for us there is none. There are many in the rest of 'normal' society who, either openly or secretly, express the view that we are quite, quite mad. But do they help us? More often, they just point at us and laugh.

Who are we? We are the Country Weekenders, city dwellers who know we belong in the woods. Shepherds and swineherds trapped inside pinstriped suits. Buxom milkmaids manacled to modular office furniture. Muddy-kneed rural urchins daily delivered in veal-crate buses to a man-made world of concrete fields and tubular steel trees.

Come Friday night, we shed our metropolitan exoskeletons and crawl, as individuals, couples or family units, into the safety of our cars. And there, as time slows down to a snail's pace, and over the course of a journey that may take up to six hours, we quietly metamorphose. We arrive in the dark, in Norfolk, Sussex, South Wales, or, in my case, Dorset, and slither quickly into bed to complete 'the change'. We wake up the next morning, and we are free. Free to grow stubble, shun Safeways, spread manure, pick daffodils and imitate the accents of the people who live nearby.

But the happiness doesn't last. Within 36 hours we start to feel the inevitable pull. The leftover risotto goes in the freezer, the holey jumpers go back in the cupboard and we go back in the car. By the time we get to Ringwood Services, we have stopped talking about dwarf French beans and sticklebacks and are making social plans for Tuesday on the mobile phone.

How do we become like this? I cannot speak for others, but I know exactly how it happened to me. Cynics will scoff at what sounds like the inevitable psychobabble confession: it all started when I was a child, and my parents were largely to blame. I was born in London, in 1965, and lived the first years of my life in a terraced house in Westbourne Grove, west London. I was a town-child. But I do have memories (and photographic evidence suggests this is no false syndrome) of abnormal exposure to organic matter: a playgroup in Ladbroke Gardens, where our mothers encouraged us to make mud pies and daisy chains; a bird table in our garden, which was itself about the size of a bird table. Once my father took me fishing in a stream in Richmond park: bamboo, string, bent pin. He 'caught' a mackerel while I was looking the other way. We took it home and ate it. I was impressed.

And then there were trips out of town, to a place called the Country, where everyone wore different clothes, and I fell in love with their dogs, slept in huge beds, played naked on cool, prickly grass, and cried when it was time to come home.

Then one day, when I was six, my parents announced that we were moving. We were going to live in this magic place, the Country, all the time. I was ecstatic. My sister, who was two years older, was confused. But we did it. We went to Gloucestershire, a hamlet called Calmsden, to live in a converted barn ('You mean real cows used to sleep here?' I loved that). Within a year I had my own patch in the vegetable garden, a box of pet snails and a collection of birds' eggs. Within two years I had a puppy.

The cunning thing about the abduction, in retrospect, was the timing. Three or four years later, I wouldn't have stood for it. By then, I would have made my pact with the urban devil, sold my soul to the Underground and the Routemaster, and considered my parents largely redundant outside mealtimes. I would have been fledged, independent, part of a west London gang, and if my parents had told me that they were moving to the Country, I would have said, 'Fine, I'll stay here if that's all right. Just show me how to cook the fish fingers before you go.'

But they kidnapped me, at the tender age of six, and I was initiated, willingly, into the cult of the Country.

Returning to London in my early twenties was exciting but obviously temporary. I had come in search of work, housing and sex, but even when I had found all three, I usually went away to the country at weekends (sometimes taking the sex with me – it being so much better in wide open spaces). After a few years, my flirtation with city life had become problematic. The cynical dalliance looked in danger of becoming a steady commitment. Still, I was able to see my true love every weekend . . . and, like a fool, I ignored the problem. Ten years later, the pathology was full-blown. Like it or not, I was a dyed-in-the-woolly-jumper Country Weekender.

This was the life I led until last year, when I decided to take the Cure. It is simple enough. Like the transsexual who gets the snip, then wears the stockings and the make-up all the time, the Country Weekender just has to make the Move; to give up playing at country life on Saturdays and Sundays and start working at it, all day, every day. Then he or she can grow vegetables, bake bread and wipe the muck off their own fresh-laid eggs until the end of time. It is what we all dream of. But few of us ever act on those dreams.

Last year, I acted: I took the treatment. The regular destination for my alter-rural-ego was a small gamekeeper's cottage beside the River Brit, in Dorset. I had been renting it, and weekending in it, for the best part of a year. It was late February, and uncommonly mild. The snowdrops and crocuses were overlapping with the daffodils. A woodpecker had been hammering cheerily on a hollow oak behind the cottage for the best part of the morning. My 'returning pangs', the technical term for the Weekender's regular Sunday-night cold turkey, had started already, and I knew they would be particularly bad. 'Sod it,' I thought. 'I'm staying.'

I didn't, of course. Not right there and then. I went back to London. But I had made a decision. I would organise things so that I could stay.

I did just that. I would spend from spring until Christmas at the cottage, where I would attempt to do the things I had always dreamt about: raise pigs, keep chickens, go fishing whenever I wanted. Build that smoker in the chimney. Set an eel trap in the river. Smoke those eels . . .

I would become a real downsizer, an urban escapee. Moreover, I would go public on the experience: I would make a film about my efforts to go native. Others, who had suffered as I had, would be able to take heart and learn from my experience, as I learnt, on my little patch, from the lifelong smallholders who live around me.

Nine months later, the cure is complete and the film is in the can. As of this evening, you can see what I went through. And where I am now. Yes, I kept chickens. Yes, I went fishing. And, yes, I raised pigs. And now I have three prosciutto-style hams wind-drying in the porch at River Cottage. And, like the back legs of my porcine charges – who lived, like me, in rural bliss – I'm cured!

February 1999

Spears of joy

At my parents' house in Gloucestershire, the second last Sunday in April is a special day in the kitchen garden calendar. On this day my father, whatever the weather, will trudge to the far end of the vegetable patch armed with a bundle of small white flags, get down on his hands and knees, and carry out an inch-by-inch inspection of a bare patch of earth about 15 metres by 10 metres. A sapper searching for mines could hardly be more thorough.

He is looking for the first peeping tips of asparagus spears. He won't find any, of course. Not for another week yet; possibly not for two. But he'll be out there every day from now on, scouring the ground like Poirot after a murder weapon. When the first purple-green shoot bursts through the soil, a flag will be triumphantly planted beside it. The next day another, then a few more, until the ground looks like a miniature army in surrender.

Why the flags? Two reasons. First, so that each spear, once marked, will not be accidentally stepped on. Second, so that no spear can be allowed to perform that trick of disappearing just when it ought to be ready for the pot, and reappearing days later so bushy it could house a family of crows.

The gathered stalks are carefully size-graded, prior to cooking, into three categories: thick, medium and thin. These have to be steamed for ten, eight and six minutes respectively. I have seen him agonising for minutes about whether a particular stem should be in the eight or six camp – then split the difference by giving it seven.

Of course, these days, with imports from around the world, asparagus (or Sparrow Grass, as it is known by the East End barrow boys) is available almost throughout the year. The fibrous, white-shafted giants from America, the stout saplings from Israel and Cyprus: these may do for a soup or a tart; the tips may even raise the tone of a dull salad. But for sweetness, flavour and tenderness, nothing can compare with the English garden variety in its proper season.

To be tasted at its best, even English asparagus ought really to be enjoyed on the same day as it is cut, preferably within a few hours. Cut asparagus deteriorates quickly. The natural sugar reverts to starch, and the cell walls toughen and become fibrous. If your grocer stocks locally grown asparagus, then there is a chance of finding a bunch in a decent condition. Courageous shoppers will feel free to quiz their grocer about the origin of his stock and delivery times, and co-ordinate their shopping accordingly. Examining the cuts at the base of the stem will give you some idea of how recently it has been harvested. Stems which have lost their rigidity, or whose tips are in the least dry or withered, should be avoided.

My father's cooking times are appropriate for very fresh asparagus of varied thickness, but if your specimens were cut more than 24 hours previously, a longer time may be necessary to tenderise the spears. Let your mouth, rather than your stopwatch, be the guide:

asparagus is ready when the tips are tender, but not disintegrating, and the stems are just on the soft side of al dente. It should then be served at once.

The best asparagus deserves to be a course on its own, unadorned with sophisticated technique. The traditional accompaniments of melted butter, hollandaise, or a simple vinaigrette, are hard to improve on. My own favourite presentation, equally simple, is the Italian style: provide each diner with a wedge of lemon and a small saucer into which you have poured a little pool of the very best extra virgin olive oil (Tuscan olive oil with the Laudemio label is highly recommended). Pass around a bowl of freshly grated Parmesan or, better still, paper-thin shavings of the cheese. Sea salt crystals and a mill of black peppercorns should also be on the table.

April 1993

Now that we have our own asparagus bed at home in Dorset, I have been able to take on fully the mantle of my father's obsession – though I've managed to stop short of the white flags. Having long ago got over my Italian phase, I also have a new favourite way of eating them: the lightly steamed spears become the soldiers of a soft-boiled egg. A little nut of butter and a few drops of vinegar stirred into the hot runny yolk of the egg with the tip of an asparagus spear, make a kind of instant hollandaise.

Ditch the bird for a happy Christmas

Several years ago now, largely at my instigation, the turkey got fired from our family Christmas dinner. Its dismissal from festive duty wasn't a decision we took lightly but, and I think I speak for the whole family here, it certainly isn't one we regret.

We had done everything to breathe life into the old bird. We'd spent about as much as you could on a turkey, opting for a free-range, organic, slow-grown bird, corn fed by West Country wenches and subsequently (rather than consequently) well-hung, with its guts in, for an extra gamey flavour. We'd deployed culinary tips from the great and good (the best of these: Anton Mosimann says cook the legs separately, like a *coq au vin*). We'd adorned it with the most sophisticated, souped-up trimmings: Armagnac-soaked prunes wrapped in bacon; grated sprouts stir-fried with ginger, chestnuts and sesame oil; home-made chipolatas incorporating the bird's minced liver and fresh truffles. The trimmings were wonderful. But the bird itself seemed unworthy of their flattery.

It's hard to be precise about why I felt, increasingly, that turkey was failing to deliver. It doesn't have to be bland and dry – though these pitfalls are all too rarely avoided. Yet even the juiciest, gamiest, most crisply skinned bird – of a kind I feel we've achieved at least a couple of times – wasn't doing it for me. Something was missing, and I went looking for it.

Whether you are religious or, like me, not, you may see the Christmas meal as something pretty sacred. It is a time when we are looking to feed our better selves. The food we choose to eat needs to spread love, warmth, good will, forgiveness and optimism around a large table of people who, though bonded together by varying levels of shared genes and shared history, might not otherwise choose to sit down and eat together. It needs to weave a spell of magic that suspends any disbelief in the meaning of family, and indeed in the meaning of Christmas. And although normal, sceptical service is likely to resume with the Boxing Day hangover, something of the spirit of that meal should linger deep in the unconscious, helping to keep us sane and sanguine for the next 12 months.

This is a tall order, and the mild, white flesh of the turkey, even at its best, simply isn't up to the job. What's required is something heartier, richer and more intense. What's needed is a flesh whose savour runs deep because its fats are dispersed, in fine grains, throughout the meat. Something that reveals itself slowly, through chewing, then yields completely. A meat whose surface, seared by the heat of a fierce oven, creates a flavour that is the very essence of savouriness, yet whose interior is so matured, tender and relaxed, it could be served raw, like sushi.

I said 'sanguine', and on Christmas day, I want to taste blood. It's time to bring on the beef. Not just any old beef, mind, but a massive, well-aged, beautifully marbled joint of roast beef-on-the-bone. Personally, I favour about six ribs-worth of the sirloin, with the fillet still attached on the concave side. A whole forerib would feed slightly less (though easily 12), but be every bit as good. You need a good butcher, not a supermarket, because you want to insist that your joint has been hung for at least three weeks. And it should be from a pure beef breed, not a dairy-cross (in the absence of reliable guidance from a trustworthy butcher, Aberdeen Angus is the safe bet).

I raise and hang my own beef, from Devon Ruby cattle, here on my small Dorset farm. This means I can take risks in the hanging that a high street butcher wouldn't. Last year I killed a steer on 1 November and asked my small local abattoir to hang it until mid-December. Then I chose my sirloin roast and hung it myself in a cool outbuilding until Christmas Eve. I had to trim off a fluffy bloom of mould and a few iffy bits. What was left was as good a piece of beef as I have ever cooked or tasted – ambrosia for the meat-eating gods.

Come Christmas Day, a piece of meat like this will do the talking. Meanwhile, selling the idea of beef at Christmas to the rest of the family may not be the easiest job in the world. Be ready for resistance. Here's a few marketing strategies to help you deal with the inevitable verbal obstructions.

'It's not traditional enough,' some will complain. Well it's pretty bloody traditional: roast beef, Yorkshire pudding, roast potatoes, good gravy, horseradish sauce – it's always been rated as the all-time great Sunday Lunch (or 'Roast Dinner', depending on your social origins). Just add crackers, party hats and tinsel and it shouldn't be too much of a struggle to feel festive.

'But we have it quite often anyway.' Explain that it is your mission, as a host and a cook, to take their experience of roast beef to a new level. You want one year's grace for the experiment. If they don't like it, they can vote back the Turkey the following year.

'It won't look right.' Granted, a 30-pound turkey looks pretty spectacular when brought to the table. But it also looks pretty sad when sitting on the sideboard, some hours after 20 hungry mouths have all done their worst, yet only managed to remove half a lily-white breast and a drumstick like a weightlifter's forearm. And when, if ever, have they ever beheld the spectacle of a whole roast forerib or sirloin of beef-on-the-bone, ribs arching for the sky, blackened with caramelised meat sugars, primal, succulent, and oozing pink juices? Because that's pretty fucking spectacular too.

Take the vote on the red-blooded version of Christmas dinner while the mince pies are being munched. You don't have to tell your guests that they too are full of the seasonally essential savour of good red meat. By now they should be getting the message.

Happy Bloody Christmas, everybody!

December 2001

Baby food

Why do most animals have their babies in the spring? I'm not asking this to insult your intelligence. I know you know that it's because the weather is getting milder, the food supply is on the up, and their young ones have a long lazy summer ahead of them to build up their strength and get on in the world.

But why do us humans not bother with such sensible planning? I guess mainly because we don't have to. We have such mastery of our living environments and such superb forward planning when it comes to our food supply that we can take care of our babies at any time of year. Add to that the fact that most birds and mammals aim to achieve independence within a year of birth, whereas the human infant still remains effectively helpless for well over two, and needs protection and maternal care for many years after that. In other words, you're going to have to get the wailing, wriggling things through a fair few winters anyway.

So, giving birth in the spring is hardly necessary for people. But it might still be nice. As it happens my sons Oscar (four-and-a-quarter) and Freddy (four months) were both born in March. No planning whatsoever in the first case. But second time around, we had at least a vague sense of a schedule. Marie said she'd thought it was perfect having Oscar in March, as she'd really enjoyed being a nursing mother through the summer months. Breast-feeding with the sun on her back, having a baby under the table while eating out of doors, long walks with the little wriggler in a sling in (relatively) fine weather – all that had been both practical and idyllic.

But one other thing had, we agreed, been particularly satisfying. Oscar first took a consuming interest (as opposed to a mainly mischievous one) in solid food at around four months – early July. This is the time when our vegetable garden is simply bursting with abundance. Consequently, the first foods to pass Oscar's lips (when they didn't stick to his face, hair and fingers) were not baby rice, rusks and gloop out of a jar. They were mashed beetroot, puréed peas, creamed carrots, crushed courgettes, and even, on one occasion, chopped spinach stirred into a béchamel made from mother's own milk. And all from our own garden.

I am aware that I'm in danger of sounding more than a bit smug when I say this, but it really was one of the abiding pleasures of new parenthood to see Oscar tucking into vegetables we'd grown ourselves. It wasn't just a romantic notion of family bliss, though of course that's a part of it. Nor was it mainly about food purity paranoia, though, like many parents, we worry about what chemicals may be in bought-in fruit and veg, and prefer organic produce for our kids. At least as strong as either of these two sentiments was the feeling that this was the beginning of the best possible education for a child about food – what it is and where it comes from.

Some may think it a fanciful notion, but I have not the least doubt that a child's interest in, and understanding of, food begins as soon as something, other perhaps than mother's own milk, passes his or her lips. Babies of even just a few months old get a pretty good look at almost everything that goes in their mouth. And they will be observing more than you think about where the food they eat comes from. Babies who are fed predominantly from a jar will inevitably think that food comes, predominantly, from a jar. Regularly picking vegetables with your baby in a sling, preparing them in front of him or her, and sharing the mash as you shovel it in, will make an equally indelible impression on a baby, who will quickly understand that there may be more to dinner time than opening jars.

Of course that's hardly practical for everyone. But every parent can show their children what food looks like before it gets turned into mush. Peeling a banana and mashing it on a plate is hardly more arduous than opening a jar, but it's a lot more educative.

Kids of all ages can be included, first as witnesses and then as participants, in cooking time as well as feeding time. It is an opportunity to present even the tiniest babies with a whole range of exciting shapes and colours, textures and even sounds. And for older children, starting to make sense of objects in the world around them, watching and helping as a pile of ingredients is transformed, by peeling, slicing, heating, stirring, into something they can actually eat, is a gentle practical lesson in maths, physics, chemistry, biology and language, all rolled into one.

Within a week or two, Freddy will embark on the same food adventure as Oscar did four summers ago. Meanwhile, Oscar has graduated from growing his own mustard and cress on a wet flannel on the window sill to having his own patch in the garden. He sowed the seeds, and has been watering his little garden whenever the weatherman fails to oblige. Although the spinach and carrots have some way to go, the peas are just coming good. He's not the most patient gardener, and has a tendency to rip the pods from the plants, and plunder the infant peas when they are still barely visible to the naked eye.

He loves them so much that when a treat, or a bribe, is called for, you could give him a choice between a pod of just picked peas, and a square of chocolate. I'm not saying he'd definitely go for the peas, but he'd certainly be torn.

July 2003

Give me credit

I've never liked the word 'foodie' – perhaps because if I accept that it is genuinely descriptive of a certain type of person, then I may have to face the fact that I probably am one. And then I might have to confront some questions that those of us 'involved' with food, either professionally or as passionate amateurs, would probably rather avoid. Questions like, at what point does our interest/passion/obsession become a bore? To what extent do we let that 'food thing' eat into (you see!) other areas of our lives? Is it sane to care as much as we do about what we choose to put in our mouths?

Battling with these questions is pretty futile because if one *is* a foodie (gulp!), one simply doesn't have the option to backtrack. 'I think I'll stop bothering with nice food and just stoke up on rubbish, so I can concentrate on more important things in life' is not a sentence I ever expect to either speak or hear.

Nor can we prevent food from permeating pretty much all our relationships. If I'm honest, I must admit that I use my cooking skills to manipulate almost everyone I know. I love cooking for my friends, especially on their birthdays, because I believe it will earn me their undying love and loyalty. And I may be able to get away with another whole year of being petulant and self-absorbed in their presence.

Of course the closer the relationship, the bigger the role of food in mediating it. And in foodie love and marriage, even when abilities are matched, there is never equality in the taking of responsibility – or indeed credit – for the cooking. It isn't just restaurants that have tyrannical head chefs. It's any household in the land where both people in the relationship think food matters.

So in our kitchen (which I struggle not to call *my* kitchen), guess who's the tyrant? Who generously offers his partner a 'choice' of what he could cook her for dinner, but in a manner transparently loaded in favour of what he has actually planned to cook all along? Who 'accidentally' puts the leftovers of the ratatouille that his partner cooked for lunch into the pig bucket, in case she suggests revisiting it at supper, for which he has other plans? And who adjusts every single ingredient in his partner's salad dressing the moment she leaves the kitchen to answer the phone. Me, me, and me. In our kitchen, it's all about me.

I've noted that partners of other kitchen tyrants learn to handle the outrageous balance of power in different ways. Some become falsely modest and acquiescent: 'Me? I can't boil an egg. But luckily Tom is just a genius in the kitchen. And of course he spoils me rotten . . .'. Others play the 'swings and roundabouts' card, hinting at mighty victories in other domestic arenas: 'She does what she wants in the kitchen, but when it comes to choosing the soft furnishings, I am the undisputed king'.

But my wife Marie, to my shame and embarrassment, just tells it how it is: 'I can't do anything without him interfering. I can see the physical pain it causes him when I'm slicing courgettes to the wrong thickness, or frying onions too fast. So basically, I've pretty much given up cooking.'

But I believe (because I have to), that there is an upside for my partner in my annexing the kitchen. For example, every now and again, usually when we have just come to the end of what seemed to me a perfectly robust and satisfying supper at home, she will say: 'Mmm. That was delicious. But I think maybe I could just about manage a little chocolate soufflé now.'

Don't be misled by the flattery and the mollycoddling choice of words. This isn't a request, it's an order. There is hard-wired female biology underpinning it, and there's no reasoning with such urges. I could try persuading her that a) the appropriate moment for pudding preparation passed some hours ago, when the offer of just such a soufflé was generously made, and declined; or that b) a few squares of untreated Green and Black's finest 70 per cent will surely quell the burgeoning pheromonal desire. And she might even say 'Fine. It's okay,' – in that special way which makes it so clear that the two things it most emphatically isn't are 'fine' and 'okay'.

The urge may be biological, but my obligation to fulfil it is clearly contractual. Like that rather amusing ad on the telly at the moment, it's all in the relationship small print. I am only allowed to be a kitchen tyrant, if I can show that I can be a *lovable* kitchen tyrant. The price I pay for exercising obsessive control at the hob is soufflés on demand. He who lives by the stove dies by the stove.

Of course, I have a counter-clause, which insists: 'Hugh will receive effusive praise for every soufflé, even if, owing to fatigue and the cavalier measurement of ingredients, it has collapsed like a punctured chocolate zeppelin. In fact, Hugh will be allowed to pretend it was meant to do that, so as to make it extra gooey and chocolatey.'

But then she gets me back with this nasty little rider: 'At no time is Hugh to claim that cooking for his family is anything other than a pleasure and a privilege; it may never be offered in lieu of his fair share of cleaning the kitchen and loading and unloading the dishwasher.'

How did I ever agree to that? I mean, whenever I cook for my *other* family (the ones that begat me), the contract is all in my favour: 'Hugh is a complete angel for taking over the kitchen and cooking yet another wonderful meal. He is therefore entitled to relax in front of the telly while Mum and Dad do all the washing up.'

My son Oscar (three-and-a-half) is beginning to show a flair for making almost as much mess in the kitchen as his father. To my astonishment I find I am already offering him the same terms . . .

May 2004

Lunchbox jury

Today I face one of the biggest menu-planning challenges in my life so far. It's not professional. It's personal. In fact it's more than just personal, it's a matter of blood and love. Tomorrow, my soon-to-be six-year-old son, Oscar, starts at his new school. They don't do school dinners there, sadly. Like all the other kids, he'll be taking a lunchbox in with him. I have volunteered to do the lunchbox for him. Not just for tomorrow, but indefinitely.

What on earth am I going to put in it? Well, it might not be a bad start to decide what I'm not going to put in it, EVER. For a start, there will be no chocolate bars. No Twix, no Mars, no Snickers, not even a KitKat. Why? Not because I see these products as entirely without merit. As it happens, I am partial to each and every one of them – on occasion. It isn't really the contents of these confectionery packages I have a problem with. It's the packaging itself. These massive global brands are already trying to infiltrate our schools, and claim a piece of our children's souls, via playground vending machines, spurious sports kit promotions, and the like. Am I, a parent, actually going to help them do it? Am I fuck!

The same applies, of course, to fizzy drinks – only more so. The brands are even bigger, and so cynically invasive they are almost viral. You can add to this the fact that, loaded with artificial flavourings, colourings and preservatives, and a simply stupid amount of sugar, they are unforgivably unhealthy (as opposed to a Mars bar, say, which is forgivably unhealthy). I'd no more put a can of Coke in my boy's lunchbox than I would a packet of Marlboro or a bottle of Jack Daniel's.

There will be no crisps. This, despite the fact that I believe crisps, of good quality and without artificial additives (so not Walkers then) are, in moderation, a fine and commendable food. Personally, I *love* a good crisp. And that's the problem. I'm painfully aware of just how hard that moderation is to achieve – for an adult, let alone a child. It's only in the last few years of rural relocation that I've managed to reduce my own one-time urban crisp habit of around 15 to 20 bags a week to a more manageable five to ten a month.

Besides, admitting crisps to the lunchbox is sure to deal a fatal blow to the possibility of including the nutritious and convenient potato in any other of its many guises. For the child who is used to a bag of crisps, a small tupperware box of potato salad is surely going to cause some kind of incident. Right now, Oscar has an unlikely penchant for cold, cheesey mashed potato, which could be a nice little lunchbox runner . . . provided there's no crisp competition.

Is this beginning to seem a little austere? I didn't mean to imply there will be no chocolate in the lunchbox. Far from it. There has to be chocolate in a child's life, and if there is no chocolate in school, then the child will be forced to conclude that the 'chocolate of life' is only to be found at home. I take the view that maths and spelling will easily be sufficient to convince Oscar that home is, on balance, a kinder and dearer place to be than school, and that a chocolate ban is hardly necessary to emphasise the point. On the other hand, I feel a dose that is a little less than daily is probably in order, just to keep the little fellow on his toes. So, I propose some form of chocolate in the lunchbox between three and four times a week, in irregular and unpredictable sequence.

In the absence of big-brand bars, chocolate will be admitted to the lunchbox in three distinct forms. Firstly, and always for preference, in the form of something chocolatey made by us (including, as often as possible, Oscar himself) at home. Brownies spring to mind. The fact that they double as an ideal mid-morning, post-lunch, and late afternoon reward for hard-working adults is of course a bonus.

Secondly, in mild emergencies, (such as when the adults have been working just a little too hard) the chocolate may appear in the form of pure, unadulterated squares of good quality chocolate (Oscar's current favourite is Green and Black's 'darker shade' of milk chocolate).

Thirdly – far from ideally, but forgivably, occasionally – chocolate may be present as an incidental 'feature' on a manufactured 'treat' item admitted, after consideration, for a balance of merit over mischief – specifically a lack of child-targeted brand bullying. For example, a relatively light coating on a biscuit (the kind that is in no danger of being mistaken for a heavily branded item of till-side confectionery) may occasionally sneak through. Chocolate Digestives – and not much else – spring to mind.

So that's the banned list, and the general ground rules for chocolate treat inclusion. Choosing what actually to put in, of the infinite remaining possibilities, is a whole different matter. But why not save yourself a lot of aggro and transfer the task to the junior consumer him or herself — with a little unseen adult tweaking, and the occasional outright veto, to steer them in the direction of sound nutrition?

Oscar and I have already had an initial consultation on the subject of tomorrow's lunchbox, and I must say I think it's gone well (better, certainly, than the first tie-tying practice, which nearly ended in a lynching). The proposed menu is a Tupperwared miniature smorgasbord of his current favourites, as follows:

Soft goats' cheese with breadsticks and oatcakes

Egg mayonnaise mixed with rice-shaped pasta

Two raw carrots

A few slices of Dad's home-made salami (non-swanks)

A home-made chocolate brownie

One apple

Three clementines

One plastic drinks beaker filled with half apple juice (the cloudy kind), half water

Now if someone sorted that little lot for my lunch, I reckon I'd be quite happy. Which introduces the intriguing notion that perhaps I should really be preparing double quantities of lunchbox every day, for the pair of us . . .

September 2004

Pat a cake, pat a cake

'See you in an hour or two . . .'

It's mid-afternoon, and I feel a small heave of excitement as I put down the phone, and think 'cake'. It's baking hot outside – but baking cool in the kitchen. The kids have been messing about with the puppies on the lawn, and are very sweaty and grubby.

'We're going to make a *cake*!' I yell, trying to shout them in. The timing is lucky . . . puppy fatigue has already set in. Puppies are dropped and scattered in the rush for the kitchen.

'I'll get the mixing bowl,' says Oscar.

'Hands, hands, HANDS!' I shout.

'They're not dirty,' says Oscar, seven.

'The puppies licked them clean,' giggles Chloe, nine.

'I licked a puppy!' says Freddy, three.

'Okay . . . no hands, no cake . . .'

Hands are washed. Flour and sugar are brought from the cupboard to the table. The butter alarm goes off in my head. Will there be enough soft butter in the butter dish? Or will I have to get a new pat of hard stuff out of the fridge? If the former, we'll make a Victoria sponge. If the latter, we'll make that delicious Elizabeth David chocolate cake where the butter gets melted with the chocolate in a saucepan and you add ground almonds instead of flour.

I locate the butter dish and it's got more than half a pat in it. Brilliant. 'Okay,' I announce, 'we're going to make a Victoria sponge.'

'But I want to make that chocolatey cake where you melt everything in the saucepan,' says Oscar.

'No!' shrieks Chloe. 'That's yucky! I want to make Victoria's sponge.'

'Want to make dot coms!' says Freddy. He means drop scones. Or rather, he *means* dot coms, which is what all of us now call drop scones . . .

I sense that we're on a roll, a Swiss Roll even, and anything is possible.

'O-*kayyy*' I say, beginning to visualise the creaming of butter, the melting of chocolate, the dropping of scones. 'Why don't we . . .' pause for dramatic effect '. . . make *all three*!'

The sheer recklessness of this suggestion causes a minor sensation – there is clapping, jumping and eye-rolling.

'Yummy, yummy, yummy . . .'

'. . . Chloe's going to have a fat tummy . . .'

'No, *you* are!'

'No, *you* are!'

'Me got a fat tummy already . . .'

'Okay, Oss, get a whole butter from the fridge, chop it up, and put it in this pan. Then get two whole bars of chocolate from the cupboard . . . break them up, and put them in too . . . Chloe, we're going to weigh three eggs for Victoria's sponge . . . choose the biggest you can find.' It's a job for Daddy's digital scales.

'One-hundred-and-eighty-seven grams!' she declares.

'Now we need the same of caster sugar, the same of the lovely soft butter, and the same of the self-raising flour.' Chloe unleashes her talent for precision weighing, and 187 grams of each of the four ingredients are soon laid out in four separate bowls.

She puts the sugar in with the butter, which is so soft it can be whisked, rather than beaten.

'You have to keep going till it's all light and fluffy.'

'It's hard!'

'No, it's not, it's soft!'

'I mean it's difficult!'

'Keep going until your arm hurts!'

'It hurts now!'

'Until it *really* hurts.'

'It *really* hurts now!'

'Okay, until it falls off . . .'

After another 20 seconds of crazed whisking, Chloe drops the whisk into the bowl, and does a rather good mime of her arm falling off.

'Brilliant. Now the eggs, a bit at a time . . . Okay, then hold the bowl and let Freddy have a go. Oss, how's the butter and chocolate?'

'Jolly nearly melted . . .'

'Okay, take it off the heat, and separate five eggs.'

'There's only four left.'

'They're whoppers, though – they'll do. Whisk the egg yolks with the sugar.'

'How much sugar?'

'Erm . . . about four of those big tablespoons . . .' Happily, it's a very forgiving recipe, E. D's chocolate cake . . .

Back at Victoria station, I'm trickling beaten eggs into the bowl which Chloe is holding, and around which Freddy is whirling the whisk. 'Slow down, Freddy. I'm going to add the flour . . .' As soon as it's all sifted in, Freddy speeds up again, and sends a cloud of flour puffing up into the air, into Chloe's face, and over the table.

'Freddy! No!' she shrieks. 'You're ruining it!' I put my hand on Freddy's to slow the whisk down to a gentle stir, and tip another shake of flour into the sieve to compensate for what has left the bowl. Together we witness that magic moment when the grainy, almost-curdled, butter-sugar-egg mix is brought together by the flour into a classic, time-honoured cake batter of the kind that flops easily and lazily over the whisk – and just has to have a finger dipped in it.

'That's enough! Or there won't be any left for the tins. How you doing, Oss?'

'Good. I've mixed the yolks and sugar with the chocolate and the butter.'

'How does it look?'

'Yummy! Can I add the ground almonds now?'

'Sure.'

'How much?'

'How much is in the packet?'

'It says "one-hundred grams".'

'Then you can add the lot!' Chloe's using the 'lastlik' rubber spatula to divide the sponge batter between the two tins. She makes such a good job of it that I'm tempted to weigh each tin, just to see how equal they are. But I realise that that way madness, or at least OCD, lies. So I put the tins straight in the oven.

'Now we need to whisk the egg whites, to finish Oscar's cake.' With me holding the bowl and Chloe whisking like a dervish, the transformation from translucent slime to heavenly clouds of soft white foam takes less than a minute. 'Half in first . . . folding, not stirring . . . up and over . . .' Fluffy white mousse meets sticky brown goo and for a moment the chances of emulsification look remote. But gradually the chocolate yields and the two begin to merge. 'That's it. Now the other half . . .'

'Will this be a chocolate sponge?' asks Chloe.

'Not exactly. It'll be a little bit spongey, and a little bit fudgey.'

'Is it a chocolate *funge*?' asks Oscar.

'Sort of, yes.' I'm piling it into a single, square cake tin and it occurs to me that it should cut very nicely into over-sized, fudge-like squares.

'We could call it Chocolate funge cube cake . . .' I suggest, silently asking E. D's forgiveness, as I slip the cake on to the oven shelf beside the two sandwich tins.

'What about my dot coms?' asks Freddy. The easiest recipe in the world, bar toast, we make them in the same bowl as the Victoria sponge, without even washing it up. Six tablespoons of self-raising flour, two of sugar, three eggs and a trickle of melted butter. Then just enough milk till the batter will 'drop' from the spoon, into a lightly greased hot pan. A minute a side, taking it in turns to flip, and by the time the cakes are ready we've made 20 of them.

The cakes are all out, upside down on wire racks. Victoria's sponge is being fanned frantically by Oscar and Chloe, trying to get it cool enough to spread with jam. The scrunch of tyres, and the yapping of puppies, announces the arrival of our friends.

We knew they were coming, and we baked a cake. Or two.

July 2006

The following piece, intended (he said defensively) as a gentle piece of self-mockery, and a reflection on the process of getting old and becoming a creature of habit, ended up in Pseuds Corner in Private Eye *– where you may well feel it rightly belongs. People have since asked me, do you really make your tea like that? And the answer, I'm afraid, is yes. As a consequence, my family, friends and work colleagues generally refuse to make tea for me, and now I almost always have to make it for myself. Did someone say 'serves you right'?*

My cup runneth over

Now, to make my tea, I need two good-sized mugs. I boil the kettle. The hot water goes into one mug first, stays for a few seconds so the mug is heated, then goes into the second mug. The tea bag goes into the first, hot mug, boiling water is poured in to within a couple of millimetres of the top, and the two mugs, one containing brewing tea, and the other containing hot water, are left to stand. After about five minutes, the mug of brewed tea is placed in the sink, where some new hot water (freshly re-boiled) from the kettle, is sloshed into it, so it overflows by about half a mug. This is to stop the well-brewed tea being too strong. The full-to-overflowing mug is now tilted a little bit, so it spills out enough tea to allow room for some milk.

Remember the second mug, full of the hot (now not so hot, but still quite hot) water that was used to warm the first mug? That is now emptied. The tea bag is fished out from the first 'brewing' mug, and placed in the bottom of the empty 'warm' mug, where a small splash of milk is poured over it. The effect of the hot tea bag, and still-warm mug, is to take the chill off the milk – and impregnate it with a mild tea flavour. To encourage both these objectives, the mug is picked up and swirled, put down for a few seconds, picked up and swirled again, and left to stand for a short while longer. The tea-coloured, warm milk is now poured from tea-bag mug to brew mug, which is given a stir.

The resulting colour is observed. A little more milk may be necessary, in which case it will go via the still-warm tea bag mug, into the brew mug. When the colour is exactly right, I will stir in exactly one rounded teaspoonful of golden caster sugar. The tea, which is at this point is still far too hot to drink, will now be left to stand for at least five minutes, before a sip is attempted.

May 2005

And talking of getting old, there will be some *things to look forward to:*

The orchard of life

You tend to get, and give, plenty of warning about your 40th birthday. Months before it happens, you make sure it's on all your friends' radars. You're looking for sympathy, and way above aver-agely expensive presents. They're looking for – demanding – an extravagant party. You canvass opinions about venues and menus with more advance warning than a wedding. And there's plenty of time to arrange the billeting of children with grannies and nannies.

When the day comes you are surrounded by your wonderful, generous, pampering friends, who cocoon you in an indulgent cloud of fuss and presents, and share with you a staggering quantity of champagne and hard-kicking cocktails. There's dinner and cake if you can remember to eat it. You dance until dawn. It's all so lovely that even your hangover makes you smile. You are left feeling that life, if not actually deferring to the old cliché, may yet prove surprisingly tolerable for the next decade or so.

It's your 41st birthday they don't warn you about. The quiet, reflective one that nobody remembers. I've just had mine. How is it that I was not flooded with e-mails, texts and phone calls, saying 'just thinking what a wonderful amazing time we were all having this time last year'? Is it possible that my friends were not, like me, replaying in their heads every hilarious and debauched moment of it? Is the date of my birthday not now permanently etched in their brains, or at least their diaries, with a note two days previous, to 'send card and present to H'? It seems not.

Forty-one is tough. Worse than that, it's tough without sympathy. The lonely angst of ageing requires solipsistic solutions. Luckily I could, to an extent, see this coming. I knew that if my 41st birthday weekend was not to be spent wallowing in self-pity, I would need to arrange, in the absence of a life-affirming party, some seriously life-affirming presents. I also knew that, realistically, I would have to give such presents to myself.

And so I ordered myself an orchard. And we spent the weekend planting it. Fifteen little trees – mainly apples, but also gages, plums, cherries, pears – and a quince. The apple varieties have been chosen with great care, after some enthusiastic research at Dorset apple day last October. The most gastronomically exciting are probably Ashmead's Kernal, which is explosively crisp and has a sparkling, champagne-like tang, and Orleans Reinette, whose light, nutty crunch comes with an amazingly complex flavour that includes hints of honey and citrus and a rose-like scent.

The trees are beautiful things, but really still quite tiny – just whippy little saplings. They are smaller, even, than the tree that

Basil Fawlty up-roots to beat his recalcitrant car with in the Gourmet Night episode of *Fawlty Towers*. (Incidentally, though I admit it isn't crystal clear from the script, I now think it very likely that the character of Basil was meant to be 41 – the perfect age for venting one's mid-life, middle-class rage on defenceless Austin Allegros).

Now that I have my orchard, I'm feeling soothed, and the likelihood of Cleese-like rage is palpably diminishing. Of course I will have to wait a long time before they produce fruit in any significant quantity. But that's part of the whole psychology of the enterprise. Delayed gratification has never been my thing. But now I have a reason to yearn for, rather than fear, the hastening of age. Because the older I am, the more productive my orchard will be.

Call me a weirdo, but I am already starting to map out my remaining years on the planet in relation to these trees. Every spring, from here on, I see family picnics beneath the canopy of blossom – albeit that for the first few years we'll have to crouch or lie down to be beneath that canopy. By the time my youngest (Freddy, age two) and his friends are big enough, and naughty enough, to be interested in scrumping, there should be fruit enough to allow for this traditional form of fruity taxation by the young. (Until then I'll have to make the orchard a no-scrump zone for Oscar, six, and Chloe, nine.) And by the time I celebrate my 50th (which I hope will be right up there with my 40th) I reckon I should be able to eat at least one item of fruit from the orchard on every single day of the year, between the middle of July and Christmas Day (allowing for correct and careful storage of the right apples and pear varieties).

Perhaps one day I will have grandchildren of tree-climbing age, by which time my trees should be big enough to welcome them into their branches. And, if all goes according to plan, I see my aged self, some 40 years from now, swinging in a hammock between the Concorde pear and the Stella cherry, waiting for shiny ripe red fruits to drop into my mouth. Perhaps I'll even pass away peacefully in my sleep, before the swaying hammock comes to a complete stop. Less romantically, I suppose I might choke to death on a cherry stone. Either way, I wonder if I'll have the wit to say 'Pip, pip!' just before I croak.

January 2006

A Slow Hand

Seasonal, local, organic, wild
– in search, and praise,
of those who do
things properly

Locally produced to die for

The following conversation actually took place in my house, albeit in French. My parents-in-law came to stay with us recently and, as ever, were laden with fine produce from their native Sologne, in the Loire Valley. They hadn't been in the house five minutes before this exchange occurred:

Father-in-law: We've brought you a foie gras terrine. We think it's the best one from around us. It's made by Monsieur Trottignon [not real name] from his own geese. He's a lovely man, but tragically his son committed suicide last week. It's very sad . . .

Mother-in-law: . . . And of course we are a little worried that the terrine may not be up to his usual standard, because we don't know whether he made the terrine before or after the son killed himself . . .

Father-in-law: I think it's very unlikely he made it afterwards. He would have taken a few days off . . .

Mother-in-law: Yes, but I bought the terrine a couple of days after the funeral, and he was already back in the shop . . .

Father-in-law: . . . He is very dedicated to his art . . .

And then, later, as we eat the foie gras, the conversation resumes . . .

Mother-in-law: It is very good . . . one of the best . . .

Father-in-law: His wife still feeds the geese the traditional way, by hand, massaging their throats to help the grain down.

Mother-in-law: They are not afraid. They come to her willingly.

Father-in-law: . . . Superb. I'm sure that he made it before the suicide . . .

Mother-in-law: . . . or perhaps he made a big batch for the wake, and this one was left over. You can be sure he would have given it his best shot for his son's funeral . . .

Father-in-law: Good point!

Me: Why did the son kill himself?

Mother-in-law: I didn't like to ask . . .

I considered introducing the thesis that perhaps the son felt his father was putting his work before his children, but in the end I felt it would be a disservice to such a surreal conversation to attempt to bring it back down to earth. And besides, the subject of the conversation was emphatically not the suicidal son, but the superb terrine. To probe further would have been to look the gift horse in the mouth, and I didn't want to seem ungrateful.

This conversation may seem stilted and unlikely in English, but you can be assured that in France similar exchanges are happening all over the country thousands of times a day. In any small town the merits and foibles of its artisan food producers are hotly debated to the nth degree. Does Monsieur Bardin put horsemeat in his sausages, and if so, is that why they're so good? Has Madame Jaboulet lost attention to detail with her patisserie since she took a lover? Furthermore, consumers are more than ready to act on such nuances. My wife's mother thinks nothing of going to one boulangerie for her baguettes, another for croissants and pain au chocolat, and a third, in a completely different town, for its legendary *religieuses*.

I don't want to labour the point any further, because I know how tiresome it is to be lectured about how far ahead of us the French are when it comes to food. God knows it's happened to me often enough. And one of the reasons it's so irritating is that it is quite clear to any food-aware visitor to France that the bland homogeneity of supermarket culture is rapidly taking its toll over there as it is over here. The frequency of such eccentric food-related chatter is no doubt declining as the artisans who provoke it are going out of business.

Nevertheless, what seems to remain at the heart of French food culture is the notion that one of the vital ingredients for all good food is a good story. This stems from an understanding that food at its best is an expression of individual differences and personality. Fine food is the product of people who care, and people who are passionate about anything are often eccentric. The gossip that surrounds them, however absurd it may sound, is a vital mark of quality.

The reason I bring all this up is not to reinforce our sense of our own inadequacy – quite the opposite. It's because I'm beginning to dare to hope that in Britain the number of such foodie eccentrics – artisans if you prefer – may actually be quietly on the increase. Around these parts it is certainly the case. In the three years since I moved full time to West Dorset I have seen dozens of local small food businesses spring up, including a fantastic small smokery, several brilliant cheese makers, a lovely soup business, a crisp business (using only locally grown potatoes), a cake and biscuit enterprise and even an award-winning organic pastry maker. Within a 20-mile radius of here, I have witnessed the opening and/or expansion of at least six farm shops, and several fruit and veg box delivery schemes. Regular farmers' markets and one-off local food fairs are undoubtedly on the increase.

All that's required to support and sustain such a healthy trend, apart from our continued and committed custom of course, is the right culture of gossip and intrigue. So, just to get the ball rolling, I'd like to tell you all that one of the partners in the crisp business is a cross-dresser, and that the smoker and his wife share a bed with their dog. Meanwhile, the soup maker has a local white witch come round and perform a spell over every batch, and the reason the organic pastry is so good is that the women who make it always sit on it for ten minutes before rolling it out. As it happens, only one of the above statements is actually true (and I have the photographic evidence to prove it). But I won't tell you which one it is, because I wouldn't want you to think the others are any less deserving of your attention. They are all excellent.

February 2004

Wild in the woods

At the end of a farm track off the A264, just a few miles from Gatwick, I encountered a scene which took me back in time: wandering among broken branches and fallen leaves on the edge of a patch of woodland, the fur bristling on their dark backs, their snouts snuffling for roots and berries in the mud, were a group of rather contented looking animals, clearly porcine, but definitely not pigs. One particularly large beast looked up from his foraging, revealing two formidable tusks pointing skyward from his lower jaw. He looked every inch a wild boar, and I was glad there was a fence between us.

In fact, he was a farmed wild boar, if that's not a contradiction. He was also, the farmer in question assured me, not at all dangerous – 'unless you get between him and a sow he's got his eyes on'.

The farmer was Harry Calvert, who started Holmbush Wild Boar Company in 1988. What possessed him to do such an eccentric thing?

'It was a combination of an act of God, rhododendrons, and a timely phone call,' he told me. The act of God was one that few Sussex farmers are likely to forget: the 1987 hurricane. It blew down a lot of Calvert's trees, and flattened one young plantation completely. 'After that we got a terrible rhododendron problem – it's amazing how they can encroach. I discovered that pigs were good at getting rid of them, roots and all, so I advertised for a few breeding sows. Then someone rang up and suggested wild boar. I was intrigued.'

He now has almost 200 animals, which is enough to sustain a regular take off. The meat is sold direct to restaurants and, through Holmbush's own farm shop and a number of specialist butchers, to discerning gourmets.

The boar are looked after by one David Williams, whose bush hat and pony tail suggest a cross between Crocodile Dundee and a New Age traveller. In fact he is, according to Calvert, 'one of the best stockmen I've ever come across'.

Dave is entirely unfazed by the boar's reputation for fierceness. When I approached a group, a young male snorted a warning, but once I had taken a few steps back, the same animal was taking pig nuts out of Dave's hand. 'I think they're a little bit smarter than domestic pigs,' explained Dave. 'They're certainly tougher. I just make sure that they have plenty to eat, and they pretty much look after themselves.'

But the boar-farming industry is having its tusking problems. For a start, not all the meat labelled wild boar in the shops is the genuine article. After my visit to Holmbush I spoke to Dr Derek Booth, secretary of the British Wild Boar Association (BWBA), an organisation set up to promote the true British boar and root out boar frauds.

'The problem is,' he explained to me, 'that the wild boar readily hybridises with the domestic pig. The cross-bred product, which is really only another type of pork, is being sold as wild boar. People who try it may be disappointed by its similarity to the pork they are used to, and will certainly resent the extra cost. Another problem is with imports of frozen wild pig from Australia – the so-called razorback, which is really just a feral version of the domestic pig. Unscrupulous game dealers in Europe are selling it as boar, but again the taste is completely different. This kind of misleading labelling is very unfair on those farmers who produce the real thing.'

Holmbush's boars have the blessing of the BWBA, though impure stock was initially a problem, as Calvert explained: 'We bought our boar as an up and running herd, and we noticed straight away that some of the stock were not as pure as they should have been. But we got rid of the iffy ones straightaway, and selective breeding since then has brought our purity to over 90 per cent.' Anything over 85 per cent is considered pretty good going, and earns the approval of the Association.

If the problems of raising boar have been largely overcome, the problems of selling it are just beginning. Until recently the only PR agents in this country for wild boar as a gastronomic treat were Messrs Goscinny and Uderzo (in translation). No Asterix book was complete without a boar hunt, and the traditional ending of rabble-rousing, roast boar-laden feast, at which Obelix in particular gorged himself stupid. But for Elsiedale Armstrong, who markets wild boar and its products for Holmbush, the 'Obelix factor' has been more a hindrance than a help.

'For most people,' she explained, 'the image of boar is of a ferocious hairy creature charging through wild woodland. The corresponding association for the meat is that it is going to be tough, sinewy and strong tasting – perhaps even rather nasty. Even when it appears on the menu of a first class restaurant, it is seen as a man's meat – something to be ordered by the macho and hairy-chested.'

This is a particular hindrance when it comes to persuading the supermarkets to stock boar meat. 'It isn't yet a product they feel comfortable with. They have started to be a bit more adventurous – most of them now sell game, including venison. But it seems that boar is just too big a leap at the moment.'

The other problem, of course, is price. It takes 14 months to 'finish' a boar for the market, as opposed to four or five for an intensively farmed domestic pig. Even then the dead cleaned-out weight of a boar carcass is a maximum 130 pounds, some 30 or 40 pounds less than most domestic breeds. 'But you can't hurry it,' Armstrong told me, 'and more intensive rearing would spoil all the natural character of the meat.'

Time is money, and the wholesale price of boar is more than twice that of pork. 'And the way the supermarkets cut and trim their meat makes it even more expensive,' said Armstrong. 'Waitrose, for example, have shown a lot of interest in our boar. But they can't figure out how to get their margins. Here at the farm shop, all out-trimmings can become something: we make sausages, pâtés, and a pie mix. But the supermarket will only sell neatly packaged, well-trimmed prime cuts of meat, because that's what the consumer demands.'

For the moment the main outlet for Holmbush's boar remains the restaurant market, and specialist high street butchers who, unlike the supermarkets, have a real appreciation of the product, and the time to explain wild boar to their customers.

But Calvert is convinced that a breakthrough will come, sooner or later: 'Look at what happened with venison,' he says. 'Ten years ago, it was a highly specialised gourmet product with a very limited market; now you can buy it in the supermarket. I believe that with wild boar we have an even better product – it's only a matter of time before it catches on.'

I certainly wasn't going to leave Holmbush without a sample of boar meat with which to make my own assessment of its chances of catching on. The farmshop's resident butcher Mark Seale was as helpful as he was enthusiastic. 'You can mature boar meat like beef,' he explained. 'There's a carcass here that's been hanging for nearly three weeks.' In the end I took a boneless leg from the well hung carcass and, on a last minute whim, a whole head from an animal that had been slaughtered just two days before. 'It makes a lovely brawn,' I was assured.

Braised gently on a bed of sliced onions and carrots, with red wine, juniper berries and caraway seeds, the leg emerged succulent and tender. My various guests pronounced it 'much tastier than pork', '. . . rich and slightly hammy . . . delicious', 'surprisingly tender' and, briefly but emphatically, 'fab'. I concurred with all of these.

I decided to entrust the head to offal enthusiast Adam Robinson, chef at The Brackenbury Restaurant near Shepherds Bush. He made it into a terrine ('I could call it brawn, but it might not have sold as well') which I ate at the restaurant the following day. Served with a piquant relish, in which juniper was again a feature, it was quite delicious.

There was one other bit of the boar's anatomy I sampled – and now I have an answer to the question 'what is the most exotic thing you have ever eaten?' Coated in flour, fried in butter, and served on toast with a squeeze of lemon, wild boar's brains are one of the tastiest delicacies I've had in ages. And I'm not just saying that to be macho.

June 1992

Shelling out

Only the heavily salaried can afford to go to work on an egg these days. A gull's egg that is. At around £10 for six, they are ten times the price and about half as big as size-four hens' eggs.

'Worth every penny,' said the besuited young banker I met buying them in Selfridges. Every penny of £1.60 each, that is. 'The flavour is unique,' he told me. 'Very rich, and slightly fishy – but fresh, like shellfish.'

I'm not quite sure I can see what all the fuss is about. At least, I think I can see it: I'm not so sure that I can taste it. For the appeal of gulls' eggs is, in my view, largely visual.

The egg, varying from sky-blue to misty grey-green, and blotched with chocolatey brown, is certainly an eye-pleaser. Nor is its beauty merely shell deep. Peel a lightly boiled (two-minute) egg to find the pearly opalescence of the white, and the deep sunset orange of the yolk. Scramble a few (three per person) and the rich intense colour is enough to stimulate any palate to the anticipation of pleasure. Add to this the indubitable aphrodisiac of price, and perhaps the gourmet's excitement can begin to be understood.

Those who gather gulls' eggs remain somewhat bewildered by the gastronomic palaver. Eggs have been collected and eaten locally for centuries now – a free and nutritious feast for those who were prepared to scout the salt marshes of East Anglia and the Solent, and bear the squawking, serial molestations of the aggrieved parents.

But elevation to the gourmet's table, and the turning of a tidy profit by professional dealers, is a relatively recent phenomenon. 'I like them,' said a second-generation collector from the Solent, 'but the difference between a gull's egg and a hen's egg seems marginal to me.' 'Marginal to the tune of £1.50?' I asked him. 'They're never selling them for that!' he exclaimed. In fact the price has come down since the beginning of the season (mid-April) as availability has increased. Selfridges is now giving away gulls' eggs at 99p a throw. It turns out the collectors sell the eggs for a mere 9p each.

I'd like to pass on the name of my collector friend, so that you can give gulls' eggs a whirl without taking out a mortgage, but he didn't want me to print his name, and refused even to be photographed for this article. For the price of gulls' eggs is high in trouble as well as money.

In Victorian times, and up until the Second World War, it was plovers' eggs which were the *sine qua non* of the society picnics of the early summer season. So avidly were their nests plundered that by the fifties the plover was deemed a threatened species, and in 1954 the collecting of its eggs was made illegal. The black-headed gull was groomed and marketed to fill the space.

'This is a very controversial business,' explains the collector, 'especially the last couple of years. It's the "antis", you see. The problem is, they think every egg we take amounts to a dead gull.'

It is a belief that has led to some unhappy incidents. One dealer decided to get out of the business this year – he was fed up of having the tyres on his car let down by antis. Another, still in business, had 'BIRD KILLER' daubed on his van in red paint. Fortnum and Mason, that epicurean Mecca on Piccadilly, no longer sells gulls' eggs. According to a press officer, 'there have been accusations of illegal taking of eggs, and complaints to the RSPB. Right or wrong, we don't like to be associated with that.'

The collectors feel the protests are founded on ignorance, and perhaps a knee-jerk reaction to a trade which seems to exist only for the benefit of an elite. 'In fact,' explained the Solent collector, 'we look after the nesting sites very carefully. The gulls are like chickens: they continue to lay until you stop taking their eggs – one egg every two days. We take each egg as it appears, leaving any nests with more than one egg in it as they may have been partly incubated. We stop collecting in plenty of time to allow them to raise a clutch. Then they will lay three or four eggs and sit on them until they hatch.'

The husbandry of the gull colonies is undertaken in consultation with the Department of the Environment in Bristol, which issues licences annually to approved collectors. Locally, the operations are overseen by conservation officers.

James Venner, of English Nature, looks after a large gullery on the Beaulieu estate, also on the Solent. He believes that the collectors' intervention actually does more good than harm. 'All they are really doing is delaying the hatching of a brood by a few weeks. This is very much in the gulls' interest, as early broods have a tendency to be washed out by the high springtides.'

Venner is empowered to deal severely with unlicensed collectors. The Wildlife and Countryside Act of 1981 imposes a fine of up to £2,000 for the theft of wild birds' eggs. And that's per egg. In the light of that possibility, perhaps Selfridges is offering a bargain after all.

May 1993

Wild time in the New Forest

I know a few strange people who actually like clocks-back Sunday. They take a perverse pleasure in the sudden winterisation of our days, get their coats and scarves out, and start smiling again for the first time since March. Some of them are crass enough to regard the extra hour under the duvet as 'a lovely little treat' – as if one hour in bed could compensate for 152 hours of daylight robbery.

I will never understand this hatch-battenner's mentality. It's not that I hate winter. I have a coat too, and I can cope. But I would rather the passing of the seasons was achieved through natural grace – not thrust upon us by some busy-body bureaucratic edict.

But I don't like to whinge. Not for too long, any way. To stave off depression, I look for compensations. They are to be found in a corresponding seasonal approach to the pleasures of dining out. Now that it is cold and dark outside, restaurants, even in London, feel warmer and more soothing on the inside. In Soho, for example, there is less of a buzz on the streets, but more of a thrill to be found behind the glass and bricks of its restaurants and cafés. In the country, a long walk on crunching grass, perhaps picking the last of the sloes, may be followed by a late lunch, when the low sun streams through the windows to warm your face and blind your eyes as the coffee arrives.

Sensible chefs follow suit on the menus they offer their acclimatising clientele. Out goes the seared tuna and light summery salsas, the ubiquitous garnishes of rocket and mache, the ice cream. In comes the oxtail and offal, darkly reduced sauces, and fat nursery puddings with an almost visible Ready-brek glow. The rocket can now be made into soup.

One restaurant that comes magnificently into its own at this time of year is the Old Manor House in Romsey, Hampshire. Here chef Mauro Bregoli serves pleasingly authentic country Italian cooking at any time of year. But come November, his trencherman's coat goes on over the whites, and he starts to cook what he loves best, with irresistible Bachannalian zeal. There are gnocchi, fat and soft, home-made Italian charcuterie, wild mushrooms from the New Forest, and a larder full of local game. Mauro is a great enthusiast for the British wild larder, and much of what's on his menu has been killed or gathered by his own hand. But, more importantly than that, he knows exactly what to do with it. It's in his blood.

I was working in Southampton last week, and finished around nine. Most of the crew, poor fools, pleaded fatigue, and headed for the local pub. But Louise, our production assistant, was game for some game, so the two of us hopped in a cab, and headed for Romsey. We arrived just before ten, as most of the other diners were getting their coffee.

'The grouse is very high,' Mauro's Scottish wife Esther told us, 'but the partridge is a bit milder, if you're not in the mood for maggots. And Mauro's very pleased with his roe deer fillet. It's become a bit of a speciality.' There was also pike: the first time I had seen it on a menu since I had *quenelles de brochet, sauce écrevisse* at the Four Seasons, when Bruno Loubet was cooking there about eight years ago. Mauro's son had caught the pike in a carrier of the River Test the previous day, so I really had to have it.

But I started with Mauro's home-made *cotechino* – an Italian boiling sausage made from local pigs, a cross between wild boar and Hampshire blue. It was richly hammy, with a lovely lip-sticking gelatinous sheen, and came with creamy, nutty lentils. With the first couple of mouthfuls my palate felt the lack of a *salsa verde*, that garlic and green herb elixir which the River Cafe would have served with this dish, to cut the fat and spice up the lentils. But then their *cotechino*, decent though it is, is not home-made. Soon I gave myself up to the unadulterated marriage of salty pig and mealy bland pulses, a pure and peasanty harmony.

Louise was purring over a plate of potato and spinach gnocci, minimally bound by flour and egg, so that they were as soft as they could be without actually falling through the prongs of her fork. They were bound with a buttery tomato sauce that was full on, without being too rich, and leant the dish a sparing dash of the residual warmth of late summer.

My pike came in a huge slab of fillet – the fish had weighed 17 pounds– and was served, skate wing style, with a caper sauce. Pike is a fish whose culinary potential has been sidelined by a reputation for vicious and near irremovable small bones. I didn't encounter a single one in my piece ('a little trick', Mauro told me later, 'I'll show you sometime . . .'). The meat was exquisite, almost bass-like in its richness, but with the clean-river taste of the best wild trout. I hope for the sake of future diners this winter that Mauro's son's luck, or skill, continues to deliver pike to his father's kitchen.

Louise had been steered firmly by Esther towards the fillet of roe deer – and had no regrets. It had been beaten flat, and pan-fried in a little butter for just a few minutes. It came with a little pile of spiced fruits and caramelised onion, which she hardly touched. 'I can't remember eating a piece of meat,' she said, 'that tasted so good on its own that it needed nothing more.'

We shared a crème brûlée for pudding, made extra nursery by the addition of bananas to the custard. I don't really go for the mucked about versions of this classic pud, but the two or three spoonfuls I managed spoke reassuringly to the child in me, and the rest was gleefully demolished by Louise.

The next morning we had a late start, and I got a bit of a lie in. The cold November air was snaking in through the open window of my rather grisly hotel room, and it chilled my nose as I dozed. But it was Mauro's cooking, not the duvet, that kept me feeling snug inside.

November 1997

Mauro is a wonderful man, and I will forever be in his debt, for it was he who first showed me how to make salamis, and instilled in me a determination to one day keep my own pigs.

Crème de la crème

What single dish would you choose to be your last? It's a question that would have many foodies I know in paroxysms of indecision. Not me.

The answer is crème brûlée, no contest. The combination of the hard crack and irresistible burnt flavour of the caramel top, with the silky, semi-set custard beneath, is one of the all-time greats.

I order a lot of crèmes brûlées in restaurants. I enjoy most of them – a good one is not that hard to make. But if I am about to exit this world for the next, a perfect one is what I would like to take with me.

And that's a more elusive creature.

First let's get to grips with the custard. Any half-decent chef knows that this should contain only four ingredients: egg yolks, sugar, double cream and vanilla pod. But there are several ways of combining these. The 'safe' method is to scald the cream with a split vanilla pod in the pan, then pour it over the beaten yolks and sugar, whisking all the time. The custard is gently cooked until it starts to thicken, then transferred to the pots in which the brûlées will be served. These are then baked in a tray of hot water to set the custard.

This technique produces a reliably set texture, but not the perfect, thick-but-ever-so-slightly-sloppy consistency that I think we should be striving for. This can only be achieved 'the risky' way, in which the custard does not go in the oven at all, but is cooked over the hob for as long as you dare, stirring all the time. As soon as it shows signs of setting at the edge and bottom of the pan, it is removed, and strained into the serving pots.

And what about the all-important brûlée? Some chefs – Alastair Little (who incidentally makes a perfect custard) and Peter Gordon of the Sugar Club – prescribe the use of Demerara sugar. It's true that it makes life easier for the chef, as Demerara has a lower melting point. But the flavour is wrong – Demerara has a distinctive note of molasses, a contamination of the pure taste that is achieved by burning a refined sugar.

No, it must be caster. The layer should be between one and two millimetres thick, and completely caramelised.

The perfect topping is a dark variegated golden brown (not black), and hard as glass.

There is also the question of timing. Some people (again, Alastair Little) like to brûlée the sugar immediately before serving which means the caramel and the top few millimetres of custard will still be warm when you eat it.

Wrong again – I don't enjoy the warm-mouth feel of the first couple of spoonfuls and the caramel doesn't have the essential hard crack that makes breaking it such fun.

Ideally then, the crèmes should be brûléed about half an hour before serving, and returned to the fridge to cool completely.

I have heard last-minute burning defended on the grounds of authenticity, because 'that's what they do in France'. But despite its French name this is probably not a French dish at all.

Escoffier has no recipe for it and even today there is no mention of crème brûlée in France's culinary bible, the *Larousse Gastronomique*.

So where does it come from?

Nobody seems to know for sure. I think of it like so many custard-based dishes (trifle, custard tarts) as quintessentially British. Constance Spry describes it as 'a speciality of Trinity College Cambridge' and the college is, to this day, proud to be associated with the dish. They don't claim to have invented it, but they do, I am happy to say, concur with most of my above prescriptions. In summer they serve their brûlée with fresh raspberries, 'the only legitimate embellishment'.

The Trinity brûlée, raspberries on the side, seems very close to perfection.

Except that these days fear of listeria means they no longer use fresh egg yolks, but substitute pasteurised 'liquid egg yolk'.

For a condemned man, that really won't do.

September 1997

Authentic, traditional, artisan – these are the vital buzzwords that get the juices flowing for those in search of real, slow food. But with the value associated with such genuine provenance ever on the up, the unscrupulous hijacking and spurious application of such epithets becomes inevitable, and they start to lose all meaning.

One product that is definitely 'not what it once was' is smoked salmon. At its best, it will always be an utter delight. At its worst, it is no better than Bernard Matthews' turkey ham. In other words, a disgrace. Caveat emptor.

Smoke signals from across the border

If the best caviar comes from Russia and the best foie gras from France, then where does the best smoked salmon come from?

The knee-jerk response of the average amateur gourmet would be 'Scotland' – and this is the answer that Norman MacLean, secretary to the Association of Scottish Salmon Smokers, would most like to hear. 'Salmon has been smoked in Scotland for years,' he says, 'and the Scottish product is the genuine article.'

A fair marketing point, and not a very controversial position, you might think – unless, like Michael Henriques of the Coln Valley Smokery in the Cotswolds, you happened to be smoking salmon outside Scotland. He feels that the marketing strategy of the big Scottish smokers is misleading, if not dishonest, and that the seal of approval of the ASSS should not be taken as sure indication of a good product.

'The ASSS is a propaganda organisation whose aim is to put it about that only smoked salmon from Scotland is actually any good,' says Henriques. 'I concede that for a long time the Scots must have been preserving their catches of salmon by salting and kippering, which is a hot-smoking technique, but the sophisticated taste that has always been appreciated by the gourmet comes from a cold-smoke technique which the Eastern European Jewish émigrés brought to London in the last century.'

Henriques, whose own smoking kilns are 'exact copies of the old London smokeholes', particularly objects to the Scottish smokers' liberal use in marketing literature of that much abused epithet 'traditional'. He cites the high-tech equipment used by the big Scottish salmon smokers, in particular a patented piece of equipment called the Torry kiln.

'It's modern, clinical and mechanically controlled,' says Henriques.

'The fish are laid horizontally on perforated trays, and the smoke is circulated by an electric fan. You just don't get the same taste as from the traditional method – allowing the smoke to curl up from the floor through vertically hung fillets, tail to head.'

MacLean does not accept this view. 'What we mean by "traditional" is that some of the ingredients and/or practices derive from a heritage handed down from generation to generation – like the recipe for the brine, which might include rum, or the length of time for which the fish is smoked.

'The truth is that anything really traditional in terms of technique probably wouldn't pass modern hygiene standards.' As for the alleged superiority of the Eastern European smoking tradition: 'It's not an argument I was aware of.'

One man who is aware of it, and indeed practises it, is fourth-generation salmon smoker Marcel Forman, of H. Forman & Sons. His great-grandfather was a Russian Jew who came to London in the nineteenth century.

'He set up a smokery in Stepney Green, which was a Jewish ghetto in those days,' says Forman. 'The smoker's art has been in my family for generations. I have learnt that it is a lifelong art. You can't expect good results just by putting a million or two into a modern plant.'

Forman is keenly aware of rivalry from over the Scottish border: 'The Scottish smokers have always attacked anyone who was outside their association. But in my view their marketing is based on selling a pack, an image, and not on selling a quality product within that pack.'

Britain's biggest producer is Pinneys of Scotland Ltd, which was established in Scotland in 1976. Its packs carry the ASSS's badge of approval and flashes of tartan; its brochure refers to 'traditional Scottish craftsmanship' and 'our age-old secret of the smoker's art'.

The really useful thing about a secret, of course, is that you do not have to reveal it. There are very few rules, or even guidelines, governing the use of terms such as 'age-old' and 'traditional'.

Pinneys' marketing director, Andrew Calvin, admits that the company does not use old-style brick kilns, but defends the wording: 'Our technique is old in terms of type of wood, length of time the fish is smoked, and the amount of smoke to which the product is actually subjected. It's a recipe which has been developed over a number of years.' Presumably since 1976, before which Pinneys was smoking salmon in Suffolk.

In terms of sales, the Scottish smoked salmon producers undoubtedly have the upper hand. But as the international market continues to expand, smokers such as Forman and Henriques are determined to undermine the perception that Scottish is best.

Henriques, throwing down the gauntlet, says: 'A nation that thrives on burnt meat and porridge can hardly be the best arbiter of subtle matters of taste.' One imagines the Scots will have a none-too-polite answer to that.

May 1992

Let's hear it for the green and hairy

What is the most patriotic of all summer fruits? The strawberry, so redolent of the English summer? Wimbledon, Ascot, Henley, straw boaters, champagne, and all that tosh? Hardly.

It's true that the only decent strawberry you'll get is an English one, in the month of June or July, but since for the other ten months of the year we are bombarded with under-ripe, gamma-rayed, curiously crunchy fruit from the USA, New Zealand, Israel, Spain and probably Outer Space, even our own truly seasonal crop seems to have lost its magic.

The raspberry might be another contender: for me it beats the strawberry for flavour every time. But the rest of Europe has as much claim on the raspberry as we, as indeed does the USA, where much of the work on improving the quality and yield of raspberry canes was done at the beginning of this century.

For me the outstanding candidate is the gooseberry. It's one of the very few fruits you won't find anywhere out of season, and which, when you do find it, is almost sure to have been grown in this country. We hardly import any gooseberries, and you rarely see gooseberries in France – a fact which some might take as extra incentive for making this a flag-waving fruit for Britain.

In Dorset the gooseberries are going down a storm. People are staggering back from the pick-your-owns under piles of the little green gobstoppers. Punnets are stacked by the till in the local Spar, catching the eyes of shoppers who apparently just went in for a pint of milk and a loaf, or a six-pack and a bag of crisps: 'Ooh, goosegogs,' they exclaim, as though Christmas has come early, 'better have some of them!'

But back in London a straw poll of just about anyone I happened to speak to over the last couple of days revealed that the gooseberry season has all but passed the capital by. Only two of a dozen could recall seeing gooseberries in the shops (they have been in season for almost a month now), and none of them had actually eaten any. Personally I haven't seen a single dish involving gooseberries on the menu of any London restaurant this summer and I've been getting about a bit.

It's sad to think that the capital no longer reflects the seasonality of the provinces.

The only way to reverse this trend is for consumers to shop with more attitude, and a beady eye on the seasons.

The great green gooseberry is as good a symbol as any with which to spearhead your personal campaign: the season has a few weeks left to run, and you will find that they are in the shops, including most of the major supermarkets, if you take the trouble to look for them.

Not least of the reasons you should try them is that they are sublimely delicious: especially now, at the end of the season, when they are properly ripe. It takes gentle cooking to bring out their subtle flavour, a sharp, sorrely tang with notes of strawberry and lychee.

Cooked until completely pulpy, in a heavy pan with just enough water to prevent burning, gooseberries will need to be sweetened with just a little caster sugar.

Very ripe specimens will benefit from a squeeze of lemon juice. This compote can be sieved to make a smooth purée, if you like your goosegogs pip free.

Chill, then serve with cold real custard, and thick (ideally clotted) cream. Mix in the mouth, not in the bowl, for the best of all possible fools.

It's mad not to.

July 1997

First catch your dinner

Scotland does not always get the credit it deserves for its contribution to British gastronomy. In fact, between the covers of this magazine, it tends not to get much credit for anything. So, with a thoroughly English sense of fair play, I will attempt to redress the balance.

A recent Scottish holiday provided a number of elevating eating experiences besides the fantastic lunch at The Peat Inn chronicled last week. I attribute the considerable pleasures of the food I enjoyed in the remote highlands to two factors. Firstly, the ability of gale force drizzle, hostile gradients and ankle-snaring heather to inspire primitive, raging hunger. And secondly, the revival within me of the dormant idea that whatever you're eating, it always tastes better if it's been caught/picked/shot by you. Or somebody else quite nearby.

While others were felling great stags, and hauling salmon from the river, my own contribution to the flesh-store was relatively modest: one brown trout, barely ten inches long, and so skinny it would have disgraced the fishmonger's slab. But it was fresh, local and plucked from the loch by my own fair, frozen hand. Rolled in oats, and briskly fried, it sure beat bran flakes for breakfast.

More productive than my fishing forays was the hunt for a more static quarry: wild mushrooms. Thanks to mycophile chefs like

Antonio Carluccio of The Neal Street Restaurant, the English are just beginning to emerge from a state of near total ignorance about this abundant source of fabulous free food. The Scots, it appears, have been canny about 'shroom hunting for some time. It was the landlord of the local pub who tipped me off. 'Aye, you'll find chanterelles in the birch wood at the top of the glen.' But, he added with morbid glee: 'There's another that looks just like it, mind, that'll kill a man at 20 paces.'

Armed with this warning and a small basket, I was soon searching for these peeping orange trumpets. The first fungi I discovered were not chanterelles, but large, heavy-headed *Boletus edulis* (ceps), as big as my trout and, gastronomically speaking, a rarer treat. These were soon followed by another monster cep. By the end of my hunt, I had made many gnomes homeless.

Chanterelles were also found, though not in the profusion I had hoped for, just enough to garnish my large plate of ceps (sliced and sautéed in butter, with garlic and parsley, served with lemon juice).

Mushroom hunting on the continent is a competitive sport, in which contestants rise at dawn to hunt for the overnight crop. English 'shroomers are less likely to encounter competition, and consequently more likely to discover huge hordes of fungi in previously uninvaded territory. For novices, Carluccio's book *A Passion for Mushrooms* is a must, not just for the stunning recipes, but also the very practical field guide to finding and identifying the edible and the poisonous.

Returning from Scotland, I was bemoaning the lack of pick/catch/shoot-your-own opportunities in the capital. A town pigeon could probably be bagged fairly easily but might get you in trouble with the law. It might get you in trouble with your internal organs as well. Grey squirrels abound in the parks, but there's not much meat on them. More promisingly, Mr Carluccio suggests that urban 'shrooming could be productive around now; giant puff balls are often to be seen in Hyde Park.

Probably the best source of free protein in London, if you set your sights higher than the rubbish bins, is the Thames. It may be a bit short of salmon these days but it's simply teeming with eels.

To tap London's inexhaustible supply of free eels, simply find an accessible, obstruction-free stretch of river, and fish the rising tide. You don't have to be an expert angler. A medium hook (size 2–6), baited generously with bacon and slung out a few yards into the swim, should produce results.

Thames eels should be eaten within hours, if not minutes, of their demise. They are surprisingly clean tasting, and jelly well: Gut the eel, cut into two-inch lengths, discarding the head and tail. Simmer in just enough water to cover – plus a splash of white wine or a few drops of vinegar, salt and pepper – for ten minutes. Pour the eel and juice in a bowl, and bung in the fridge. It may not be Scottish salmon, but at least you know it's wild.

October 1990

A silver miracle

Sprats must be one of the most under-appreciated delights of the English marine harvest. Here in Dorset, though, a fair few of us have cottoned on.

Sometimes the waves of the big spring tides will dump them, live and wriggling, on to the shingle beach, and those people lucky enough to be around will fill their pockets, bags, and even – quite literally – boots. The sprats also swarm into the harbour sometimes, where a drop net or throw net can be used to haul them out by the dozen.

The resulting feast is always a joy. You don't really have to gut them when they're this fresh; I usually just snip the belly and the gills so that everything can be eaten. And then I lay them on lightly oiled foil, season with salt and pepper and flash them under a very hot grill so they blister and crackle. Turned after three minutes, they're done in five. Or, in barbecue weather, I'll fire up the charcoal, thread the sprats in batches of 15 or 20 through the head on to a bamboo skewer, brush with oil and grill them on the fire.

They don't need much, sometimes just a squeeze of lemon, sometimes a little dipping sauce made of mustard, crème fraîche and a pinch of sugar. This year I tried them with my home-made plum dipping sauce. Wonderful.

December 2004

Spring stingers

The weather may have taken a slight turn for the worse, but spring has taken too firm a hold to back down now.

Walking in Regent's Park at the weekend, I noticed that the nettles are well on – about a month ahead of last year – and in perfect shape for an early spring version of one of the great dishes of the free food larder, nettle soup.

It's time, then, for you to test my theory that no one, not even in London, is more than ten minutes' walk from a bed of nettles. (Urban gatherers should, however, avoid picking too close to roads where traffic fumes will render your crop somewhat leaded.) Nettles are best harvested like tea: the crown and the top two pairs of leaves will be the tenderest and sweetest.

Pick with stout rubber or garden gloves until you have a good half-a-carrier-bagful. And if any park-keeper should challenge your actions and ask you what on earth you think you're doing, just say: 'Your job, mate.'

Here's my recipe:

Nettle soup

Serves 4

1kg/½ carrier-bag fresh nettle tops; 1 large onion, finely chopped or grated; 1 medium carrot, finely chopped or grated; 2 sticks celery, finely chopped or grated; 1 clove garlic, crushed; 50g butter; 2 rice cakes, or 1 heaped tbsp cooked rice; 1 litre fresh chicken or vegetable stock; pinch nutmeg; salt and freshly ground black pepper; 4 tbsp double cream or crème fraîche

Wash the nettle tops thoroughly and rinse in two changes of water. Sweat the onion, carrot, celery and garlic in the butter, until the vegetables have softened. Pile in the nettle tops and pour over the stock, bring to the boil, and simmer for 5 minutes until the leaves are tender and completely wilted. Add the cooked rice or rice cakes, blend the soup in a liquidiser and return to the pan. Add the nutmeg, and season to taste with salt and pepper.

Divide between four bowls, and swirl a tablespoon of cream or crème fraîche in each bowl before serving. This soup is also delicious served chilled.

March 1998

Ferry fresh

The Channel Tunnel continues to bore its way Francewards, and in a different sense around the dinner party circuits of the middle classes. Meanwhile those of us who wish to escape dinner with the bores for a quick fix of Gallic gastronomising still have the option of the cross-Channel ferry. I've just made my first use of it since I was a spotty teenager standing on tip-toe and thrusting out my bum-fluffy chin to convince the man at the duty-free check-out that I was entitled to a drop of the hard stuff (of course he wouldn't have cared if I'd been two, but we mustn't detract from these seminal adolescent breakthroughs).

Having reacquainted myself with Sealink, I'm now delighted to rejoin the Channel bores, and chip in with my comment, well-rehearsed over the last few days, that it would be a terrible, terrible shame if the tunnel put the ferries out of business. I believe this sincerely, not because I am sentimental about sailing, or because I respect the centuries-old tradition of invading France in uncouth hordes by boat. I believe it because the Sealink crossing (from Newhaven) is the only half sensible way of getting to Dieppe. And having just discovered the joys of this pretty port – surely the only Cross-Channel ferry terminal with half-decent architecture, genuine atmosphere, and serious culinary opportunities – I am keen to make a return visit.

A day trip to Dieppe is just about feasible. But with the crossing three to four hours each way, you'll be lucky to have four hours to do your tour of the charcuteries, patisseries, traiteurs, fromageries and *marchands de poissons*. A one-night stopover, however, gives you ample time to stuff your face, and stuff your bags with more things to stuff your face with when you get home.

As far as the first facial-stuffing is concerned, you could do a lot worse than eat dinner at the Marmite Dieppoise. I don't know if you could do any better, as it's the only Dieppe restaurant I was able to visit. But I've never had mussels fresher, or better-cooked (i.e. barely), in a simple, wine-rich *court bouillon*, than at this friendly, unpretentious, utterly charming restaurant. Other starters worth trying are the salad of mixed smoked fish, or any of the *coquillages*.

The dish after which the restaurant is named is also a triumph: a cream-enriched fish stew, spiked with chervil. Its main constituents were a fillet of sole, a piece of monkfish tail, and a wing cutlet of a much underrated fish, brill, which in this case really lived up to its name. I dare say the contents varies with the catch. What's obvious is that only screamingly fresh fish are allowed in, and what's rare for a dish that calls itself a stew is that none of the fish are remotely over-cooked or disintegrating. The garnish of a whole langoustine is another bonus – don't forget to eat the contents of its skull, brown meat that is sweet as a nut. Which of course it is, in a way.

Try and ensure that your day of departure from Dieppe is a market day. And don't have any breakfast in your hotel but graze instead on the fantastic produce of the market. Here, between the huge cheese caravans and vegetable stalls, gap-toothed old ladies and grey-stubbled old men with voices like gravel have set up small tables from which they sell the morning's harvest: a few goat cheeses, a box of *haricots jaunes*, a couple of rabbits, or a home-made *boudin noir* (black pudding) and a few bunches of chives.

Most spectacular, and incredible value, are the fish stalls. I brought back in an ice-box five pounds of mackerel, one of black bream, a three-pound gurnard and two dozen oysters. Altogether they cost me about a tenner. So fresh were they that I incited not a comment or a clothes peg on the way home, and even the Newhaven sniffer dogs let me pass unmolested.

So roll on roll off the ferry. Down with the Channel Tunnel. Long live Dieppe. *Y allez vite, et bon appétit.* You'll need one.

September 1991

Aga saga

In Penn, near Beaconsfield, where suburbia struggles to be all green fields, ponies and country gardens – and damn nearly makes it – there you will find Mary Berry's Aga workshops.

When I arrived for a one-day session called 'Making the Most of the Aga' I found myself the only man among 20 kitchen-proud housewives. We met, as housewives do, over coffee and biscuits, before the business of the day began. Bar a couple of loners, most of the women had, it appeared, come in pairs. Consequently they sized each other up in clusters of four and six. I homed in on a stray twosome to make a crowd of three.

'I have to confess,' said bottle-blonde Judy with topped-up tan, from Farnham, 'that cooking isn't really my thing. I'd rather be playing golf or tennis.' In Spain, she might have added, except that her 'Marbella Beachlife' sweatshirt had already made the point. 'If I do make an effort,' she continued, 'it's just not appreciated. My family will gobble up everything: for me this is just a nice day out. Maggie brought me along.'

Maggie, who seemed a demure and unlikely sidekick to her sporty friend, turned out to be something of an Aga workshop groupie. 'I've been eight times,' she told me. Wasn't 'Making the Most of your Aga' a strange one to be doing as number nine? 'Oh, I've been to this one before. But Mary told me she changed all the recipes, so I thought I'd come again.'

It turned out that practically everyone I asked had been at least once before. As we shuffled into Mary's kitchen, tea cups rattling on our saucers, I wondered just how much there was to learn about Agas. I mean, they have hot plates and ovens like every other cooker. Was it learning or entertainment, practicality or an escape from drudgery, that put so many housewives' bums on Mary Berry's foldaway canvas chairs?

There is no doubt that Mary Berry is a pro. A sprightly 60-plus, she was doing cookery demonstrations in public and on television when I was still standing on a chair to make peppermint creams.

To grab the ladies' attention, she began with a neat stunt. Announcing that the first recipe was to be a cheesecake, she put a few Digestive biscuits in a plastic bag, and tossed them nonchalantly to the ground.

A murmur of surprise rippled through the seated ladies. Mary then began to grind the plastic bag beneath one foot, like a movie starlet putting out a cigarette – she was, of course, making crumbs for her cheesecake's biscuit base. 'You need good strong plastic bags for this. That wonderful firm Lakeland Plastics does them in rolls by mail order.' This was the first of a number of plugs for kitchen products, some of which, it turned out, she just happened to be selling in the lunch break.

When it came to baking the cheesecake, Mary addressed the ladies with a cunningly divisive question: 'Now who has a four-oven Aga?' An elite minority of five tentatively put their hands up with thinly disguised glee. She went on to explain that the hot (roasting) oven of a two-oven Aga could be simply converted to a moderate oven (the baking oven of a four-oven Aga) by slotting a cold baking sheet into the top set of runners.

'You know, I've had my Aga for two years,' confided one of the loners, and a first timer, out loud to the whole group, 'and I never knew that. I always move my cakes and tarts up and down between the hot oven and the simmering oven. Of course, I usually burn them.' Sympathetic murmurs stirred around the room.

Further revelations on the taming of the ceramic-plated beast were the Aga breakfast – sausages, eggs and bacon cooked in the large roasting tin on the floor of the roasting oven – and the cunning deployment of the simmering (cool) oven to finish steaming vegetables started on the hot plate. You can even use the Aga to open difficult tins: Mary put a well-stuck jam jar upside down on the hot plate for a few seconds, gave the lid a twist with an oven-gloved hand, and hey presto!

At lunch it became clear that Maggie was not the only Mary Berry junkie in the class. 'I just wanted to say,' piped up one enthusiast, 'that your celebration cake is fantastic.' Another took her cue, '. . . and your pavlova is delicious. The recipe works every time.'

In the afternoon, Mary continued to hold the ladies (and myself) spellbound with a series of recipes well-punctuated by handy hints. 'Do you ever get a problem with condensation in the simmering oven?' asked the Aga agony aunt, rhetorically. 'It could be that the lid of your stockpot does not fit tightly enough.'

October 1993

The next three pieces are chosen from a long-running series I did for the Sunday Times *in the early nineties, on chefs and their signature dishes. I've chosen them because they are three of my favourite chefs from the series, and they happen to be three very fine recipes too.*

Fish soup opera

Inhabitants of Marseilles have two passions: football and fish soup (or *bouillabaisse*, to give it its proper name). Correspondingly, the Marseillais have two heroes: Chris Waddle, formerly of Spurs and England, now the leading Marseilles goal-maker, and the rascasse, or scorpion fish, without which no *bouillabaisse* is considered complete. Of the two, Waddle is, at the present moment, probably receiving greater attention. However, priorities will re-order themselves, and the Marseillais will be singing the praises of the rascasse long after Waddle has hung up his golden boots.

Outside Provence, only one restaurant in France produces a *bouillabaisse* considered worthy of acknowledgement by the Bouillabaisse Society of Marseilles (the Fish Soup Mafia). It is Charlot,

Roi des Coquillages, near the Moulin Rouge in Paris, which has rascasse specially brought in by overnight train from Marseilles, arriving fresh every morning.

In the face of such puritanism and snobbery, it is no surprise that English chefs almost never attempt to imitate the authentic Marseilles *bouillabaisse*. A visit to the local fishmongers is unlikely to furnish you with a rascasse, or any of the other Mediterranean rock fish generally considered *de rigueur*.

However, such is the vogue for earthy Provençal cooking, that many restaurants now offer a version of fish soup cobbled together from the best the fishmonger can provide, and almost certainly served with the traditional accompaniment of croutons, *rouille* (garlic mayonnaise) and grated cheese. Some are adequate, many distinctly watery and lacking in robust fish flavour. Probably none is as successful and well-regarded by connoisseurs as that prepared by Richard Stein at the Seafood Restaurant in Padstow, Cornwall.

Stein, the author of *English Seafood Cookery*, has the advantage of instant access to the daily catch of Padstow's fishing fleet. He also refuses to be daunted by the dogmatism of his counterparts in Marseilles. 'A lot of the talk about the right species of fish, the rascasse and so on, is old wives' tales. It's no big deal. The important thing is to use fish which have a good, strong flavour, and plenty of heavy bones. Boiling the bones gives gelatin to the stock, which helps to thicken the soup.' British fish that will admirably perform this function include dogfish, rays and conger eel, the less readily available weaver fish and wrasse and, Stein's favourite, the gurnard.

These are bolstered with cheap (but fresh) white fish, such as whiting and grey mullet. 'The other thing which I think is essential is to remove all the bones before you liquidise the soup. I've had many a soup in Provence which has a nasty bitter taste because the bones have been left in.'

As Stein dares to think he can improve on the Provençal method, he would probably be unwise to appear at a meeting of the Bouillabaisse Society of Marseilles. However, the recipe that follows will help home cooks come to terms with a dish that is, despite the raging debate, a lot easier than scoring goals for Marseilles.

Fish soup

Serves 4

5fl oz olive oil; 6oz onion, chopped; 6oz celery, chopped; 6oz leek, chopped; 6oz fennel, chopped; 5 cloves garlic; 2-inch piece orange peel; 10oz tomatoes; 2 tsp tomato purée; $\frac{1}{4}$ of a large red pepper, blistered under the grill and peeled; 1 bayleaf; a large pinch of saffron; $\frac{1}{2}$ pint shell-on prawns; salt and freshly ground black pepper; cayenne pepper

For the fish stock: 2lb (900g–1.3kg) fish such as conger eel, skate, cod, dogfish, shark (do not use oily ones such as mackerel and herring); 3 pints water; 1 onion, finely chopped; 1 carrot, finely chopped; 1 stick of celery, finely chopped

Fillet the fish and use the heads and bones to make a fish stock with the three pints of water and an onion, a carrot and a stick of celery, finely chopped. You can also use shellfish scraps, such as lobster or crab shells. (Add the cold water, then bring to the boil and simmer for 15 minutes, allow to cool before straining.)

Heat the olive oil in a large pan and add the chopped onion, celery, leek, fennel and garlic. Cook until the vegetables are very soft, which should take about 45 minutes. Add the orange peel, tomatoes, tomato purée, red pepper, bayleaf, saffron, the fish fillets and the prawns. Cook briskly, turning everything over as you do. Now add the fish stock, bring to the boil and simmer for 40 minutes. Liquidise the soup and pass it through a conical strainer, pushing as much as you can through with the back of a ladle.

Reheat and season with salt, pepper and cayenne. Serve the soup with French bread croutons, fried in olive oil, then rubbed with garlic, *rouille* (garlic mayonnaise) and some grated Gruyère cheese.

July 1991

The cook of the north

"E's done well, that Heathcote feller,' said my taxi driver in broad Lancastrian. 'Put Longridge on the map.' As we arrived in this unexceptional sprawling village, which has neither the quaintness of the rural north nor the industrial nostalgia of Lancashire's mill towns, it occurred to me that 'putting it on the map' was no mean feat.

Yet it is here in his native northwest, in a modest white-washed stone cottage, that chef-proprietor Paul Heathcote has decided to pursue his culinary ambition. After a decade of hard graft in some of the country's top hotels and restaurants Sharrow Bay, The Connaught, Le Manoir – he has gone home, and gone solo.

Against the odds – unassuming premises, off the tourist trail, high price bracket and the recession in mid-plunge – business is booming. His eponymous restaurant, Heathcote's, has become the gastronomic Mecca of the northwest.

His cooking reflects a determination, despite his illustrious tutelage, to acknowledge his northern roots, and celebrate the best of local produce. 'You can tell by my accent,' he says, 'that I'm not a foreigner. So why should I cook like one?' The point is proved on the menu, which includes dishes to warm the heart of any true Lancastrian. One starter is black pudding with fried potatoes and a poached egg, another a robust and flavourful soup of parsley and potato. A main course of beef fillet in a red wine sauce comes with a generous hunk of oxtail. 'I sometimes cook a tarte tatin,' confesses Heathcote, then adds with a glint, 'but I call it apple pie.'

The story behind one of his star dishes reveals an exceptional level of dedication to his local suppliers. Heathcote gets his chickens from Reg Johnson, a local farmer, who used to supply him at Broughton Park, a nearby hotel whose kitchen Heathcote ran before he came to Longridge. 'He was supplying us with turkeys from his farm in Goosnargh for the banqueting side,' Heathcote recounts. 'I asked him if he did corn-fed chickens, and he looked at me as if I had two heads. But a couple of days later he came back, and asked if he could have a chat. 'About these corn-fed chickens . . . I've been doing a bit of reading up, and I reckon I might have a go at breeding a few.'

The two embarked on a joint venture to create the ultimate in flavour-packed poultry: 'We made a few mistakes to begin with, and got rather a high mortality rate. We realised that the diet was so rich that the chickens didn't need so much feeding, but they took a few weeks longer to be ready. It took about a year of Reg experimenting with the breeding programme, and me cooking the birds and testing them for flavour, before we got it right.' The resulting bird, the Goosnargh corn-fed chicken, is now in demand from top chefs all over the country.

'Having achieved this,' Heathcote explains, 'I wanted to create a dish that really did justice to this bird. It had to be very simple – the flavour's so good you don't need to use any stock for a sauce.' Instead, Heathcote poaches the bird's breast in the oven, with water and a little wine. The base for the sauce is nothing more than the juices that run from the meat during cooking, thickened with butter, and flavoured with fresh tarragon. The dish is elevated with a simple garnish of asparagus spears and wild mushrooms 'I like to give the punters their two veg,' says Heathcote, 'and both of these go very well with chicken.' The punters get their dose of carbohydrate, too: little dumplings flavoured with more tarragon, and pan-fried until crispy. 'A posh restaurant would probably call them gnocchi. But I call them dumplings, because that's what they are.'

There are no frills in the name of the resulting dish, which Heathcote calls:

Goosnargh corn-fed chicken with asparagus, wild mushrooms and pan-fried tarragon dumplings

Serves 4 as a main course

4 breasts of corn-fed chicken; 125g butter; 1 dsstsp shallot or onion, finely chopped; 2 tbsp white wine; 8 tbsp water; 1 dsstsp whipping cream; 200g cooked pleurotte, porcini, or other wild mushrooms (or substitute button mushrooms); fresh tarragon, chopped; $\frac{1}{4}$ of a lemon; 12 spears asparagus, cooked al dente and refreshed in ice-cold water; salt

For the dumplings: 100g butter; 150ml cold water; 125g sieved self-raising flour; 3 tsp cooked onion, finely chopped; 1 tsp tarragon, chopped; 4 eggs

The dumplings should be prepared in advance as follows: melt the butter in the water and bring to the boil. Add flour, onion and tarragon off the heat, and beat with a wooden spoon, just until the mixture leaves the side of the pan. Allow the mixture to cool a little, then beat in the eggs one at a time to get a stiff glossy paste.

Place the mixture in a piping bag with a ¾-inch plain nozzle. Pipe 1-inch dumplings over the top of a pan of boiling water, cutting with a small knife and allowing the dumplings to drop into the water. Cook in batches for two minutes, removing each batch with a slatted spoon and placing in a colander to drain.

Seal the chicken breasts in 50g of the butter, skin-side down. Add shallot or onion, and white wine. Bring to the boil, add water, cover with a lid and place in oven at 180°C/Gas mark 4 until cooked (10–15 minutes).

Remove the chicken and strain the liquid through a sieve into another pan. Bring to the boil, add the cream, whisk in the remaining butter in pieces, then stir in the mushrooms and the tarragon. Season with salt, a good squeeze of lemon, but no pepper. Add the cooked asparagus to the sauce and warm through.

Sauté the dumplings in hot oil until well browned. Pour the sauce over the chicken breasts, then garnish with the dumplings, and serve.

August 1992

The duck that made her ladyship grouse

Disagreeing with Elizabeth David about cooking is like disagreeing with God about religion, especially since the grande dame of British cookery is now guarding the gates to that great kitchen in the sky. But the self-taught chef Stephen Bull, who runs his eponymous restaurant in Blandford Street in the West End of London, has never allowed himself to be dictated to, either by the whimsy of temporary trends or by the Woman Whose Word is Law . . .

So the fact that David, who was a not infrequent visitor to his previous restaurant in Richmond, once sent back the dish he regards as one of his best remains a source of quiet pride. For Bull is a nonconformist. He cooks what he likes, and there's no guessing what he likes until he cooks it.

The dish in question is not, unlike so many chefs' signatures, a complex creation presented as art on a plate. It is a duck, roasted whole, served with a simple gravy made from its own juices. The dish flips in the face of fashion, which currently dictates that a duck's legs should be removed, and made into a confit, while the breast is cooked separately, and served pink and bloody. Bull's duck is roasted until the skin is crispy and the leg meat cooked, by which time the breast meat is just about coming away from the bone.

'I don't like this idea that we all have to eat pink meat all the time,' explains Bull. 'There's nothing wrong with well-cooked meat, provided it is still succulent and full of flavour. And my duck has both these qualities in the extreme.' You will gather from this that the reason the late great David returned the dish to the kitchen was that it was, in her view, overcooked. 'It was ironic,' Bull recalls, 'because I was so pleased that she ordered it. In the end we had to agree to disagree.'

To produce the duck that disappointed David, but continues to delight Bull's customers, took years of fine-tuning. 'The skin is the greatest delicacy a duck has to offer, and getting the skin perfectly crispy is what this dish is all about.' Bull found it was crucial where the bird was pricked before roasting. 'You have to pierce the skin in those places that allow all the fat to run out, but not the juices from the meat.'

Another problem was the way a duck sits in a roasting pan. Usually the head end of the bird is higher up, which means it will cook too fast and be prone to drying out. Bull developed a brutal technique to overcome the problem: 'I break the duck's backbone. It's quite easily done, if you turn the bird on its breast, and apply pressure on the middle of the backbone with your fist. Turn the bird's breast up again, and it sits obligingly flat on the roasting tin.'

Apart from the gravy, for which Bull's simple recipe is definitive, the bird needs something sharp to cut through the rich meat. 'I used to do an apple and orange sauce, with very tart Bramley apples, zest of orange and a little brown sugar. It's a very good sauce, but I decided to change it, out of boredom. I tried segments of fresh lime in a light sugar syrup, and it worked so well I've tended to stick with it. The lime syrup seeping into the gravy is particularly delicious.'

To find out how delicious, follow Stephen Bull's instructions to the letter:

Roast duck with lime compote

Serves 4

1 large, fresh duck, dry-plucked, with giblets if possible (do not use a frozen duck as the skin will not crisp well and the meat is likely to be dry); 1oz butter; 1 carrot, chopped; 1 pint water or light meat stock; 1 onion, chopped; 1 stick of celery, chopped; 1 clove garlic; crushed bouquet garni

For the lime compote: 3–4 limes; 2oz sugar; 5 tbsp water

Preheat oven to 220°C/Gas mark 7. Wipe the duck, remove any bits of wax, particularly from under the legs. Remove the feet at joints and throw away. Cut off the wing tips at the second joint and chop them roughly. Cut off the parson's nose (to allow the duck to fit snugly in a roasting tin) and throw away. Brown the bits of duck and vegetable well in the butter (pour off any excess fat), add 1 pint of water or light meat stock, the garlic and the bouquet garni and cook gently while the duck is roasting.

Prick the duck well along the underside of the breast and where the legs meet the body, taking care not to puncture the meat of the breast or legs. Turn the duck over and press down on the middle of the backbone to break it. This allows the duck to sit flat in the tin and to brown evenly, breast side up. Salt the breast lightly and place in the oven for 15–20 minutes to start the fat running.

After this time, pour off the accumulated fat into a tall heat-proof jug, turn down the heat to 180°C/Gas mark 4 and keep pouring off fat and any brown juices every 20 minutes. The duck should always be sizzling merrily. Cooking time will be about 1 hour 45 minutes, depending on the size and fattiness of the bird, but more cooking to remove more fat will not do any harm. The whole point is to remove all the fat from the breast, and as much from the legs as possible.

Make the lime compote while the duck is cooking: with a very sharp knife remove all the skin and pith from the limes and either segment them between the membranes, or slice them across thinly. Dissolve the sugar in the water and let the limes steep. You can cut some of the dark green lime skin into fine strips (removing all pith first) if you wish, but blanch them for 30 seconds first and refresh, then add to the compote.

When the duck is cooked, pour off the accumulated duck fat from the brown residues, strain the stock from the combined giblets and vegetables and reduce to a gravy, skimming as you go, then add to the residues. Thicken with cornflour if necessary, slaked with red wine, port or brandy. Season. There should be four tablespoons of gravy per serving.

September 1992

Grandeur in aspic

In my last review I referred, perhaps just a mite sneeringly, to the 'gammon and pineapple school of seventies cooking'. Who'd have thought I'd be eating my words, more or less literally, so soon?

Yes, I had gammon and pineapple for lunch last week. And by God it was good. But then I did have it at an establishment in which God would probably choose to lunch — especially if he wanted to impress his friends. I had it at the Connaught.

Actually I have always liked gammon. And when I saw it was one of the two 'regular luncheon dishes' (it's on the menu every Tuesday), I could hardly not order it: when life offers you an opportunity, however slight, to share a little joke with yourself, you have to take it. I didn't know for sure it was going to come with pineapple but the admirably unfashion-conscious menu description, braised gammon California, seemed to be hinting that tropical fruits were likely to be involved.

Since I was having the gammon as a main course, it seemed only natural to start with an avocado and prawn cocktail. You couldn't say the Connaught's version is a pretty dish: it comes moulded into a large ball, served in a battered pewter cup. But you couldn't fault the ingredients: perfectly ripe chunks of buttery avocado, large Atlantic prawns and, an unexpected bonus, some flakes of poached salmon. The dressing was classic: pale pink, and almost certainly made from real mayonnaise, ketchup, Worcestershire sauce, lemon juice and Tabasco. Who would have it any other way?

My friend Ivan, an accomplished gastronome with a penchant for timeless classics, ordered *consommé en gelée 'Cole Porter'*. This was simply a bowl of rich, beefy (probably ox-taily) crystal clear jellied stock, garnished with a sprinkling of finely minced hard-boiled egg, so it's hard to see how Cole Porter got involved. Perhaps, like Ivan, he just liked it a lot.

Back to that gammon. It arrived in fine style, on a trolley (more properly called a chariot) beneath an enormous silver dome. This monumental piece of silverware was swivelled under the platter on the chariot to reveal a simply enormous leg of gammon, glistening with its coating of caramelised brown sugar and mustard. It was carved before my amazed eyes, in beautifully even slices, by a little man in a black tie who had probably been doing this for several months of Tuesdays, but never with any less care.

California turned out to spell pineapple and peaches. Both had been glazed with sugar that had been caramelised under the salamander. Done like this, the whole sweet and sour potential of the fruit was fulfilled beyond all expectations, and went very nicely with almost-too-salty, and wonderfully flavourful gammon. There was parsley sauce too: hardly exciting, this bland white sauce, flecked sparingly with the finely chopped herb. But that was the whole point of it, and the soft, milky sauce, a comforting smother to the acid, sugar and salt, actually made the dish.

The little man in black somehow made the offer of seconds sound like one I shouldn't refuse. Seconds, of course, turned out to be firsts all over again. But it was such a treat that I managed. Meanwhile Ivan was slowly working his way through a huge tureen of Irish stew: meltingly tender lamb, on (and) off the bone, in a sauce that was thickened by puréed potatoes, and had a few whole ones bobbing around among the lamb. He thought it almost a caricature of the dish: 'delicious, though I don't suppose you'd ever get one like this in Ireland. More's the pity.'

By rights I should have had Black Forest gâteau for pud, and had it been on the trolley I could certainly not have resisted. Instead I chose another enduring classic, crème brûlée. I ordered the same pudding the last time I came to the Connaught, almost seven years ago. It hadn't changed a bit. The brûlée top was made, as it should be, with caster sugar (not Demerera), and the custard was perfect: thick, but still a little loose, and speckled with the seeds of a real vanilla pod. Nestling at the bottom of the dish (the same kind of pewter cup that my prawn cocktail came in) was a clutch of fresh raspberries. I like raspberries with crème brûlée, but I prefer them served on the side, so they don't transmit their flavour into the custard. But I'd hardly expect the Connaught to change the habit of several lifetimes just for me. And Ivan wanted nothing changed about his trifle.

Simon Hopkinson and Lindsay Bareham are about to publish a cookbook called *The Prawn Cocktail Years*. This loving retrospective is sure to be a bestseller, and I've no doubt it won't be long before fashionable young chefs, who were barely out of nappies first time around, are all serving jellied tomato ring, chicken Kiev, and rum baba, all with a generous side order of ironic smiles. Provided it is done well, I expect to enjoy this timely revival as much as anyone. But it's worth remembering that the Connaught has never stopped serving this kind of food, and, because nobody does it better, has never felt the need for irony.

As Ivan pointed out, what the Connaught has, no modern retro usurper of bygone culinary elegance can ever hope to replicate. The grandeur continues to fade, but at such a geological rate that I dare to hope my grandchildren will still be able to enjoy it, just as it is today (and was yesterday). It pulls off the remarkable feat of being the most quintessentially English, and resolutely French of restaurants, both at the same time. The sheer delight of the place lies in the fact that both culinary cultures are preserved strictly in the aspic of the old school: this is a living museum of our culinary history. And just like our other great museums, the V&A, the Natural History, and the Science Museum, everybody should go there once.

Entry is not free, of course. Our lunches came from the set menu at £25 a head. Some might hesitate to call that a bargain – but for me the experience was priceless.

October 1997

It seems fitting to end this chapter, and this collection, with a memorial tribute to my old friend, Dorset lobster fisherman Dennis Cheeseman. If ever there was a man who wasn't in a hurry, who always had time for his craft, his family, his pupils and his friends, it was Dennis.

In memoriam: Dennis Cheeseman

I am sometimes asked, in interviews and by people who come on our River Cottage courses, who my culinary heroes are. I tend to say something along the lines of: Elizabeth David, for instilling in me the notion that the best food is intrinsically rooted in the soil and landscape of the region from which it comes; and Keith Floyd, for demonstrating that all good food has a people-based story, both in the production, and in the eating, and the best food television is simply the kind that tells that story with relish, good humour and respect. (Okay, I know that's a bit stodgy. Let's hope it comes across a bit more chatty in a live session.)

But we all have other kinds of hero we don't often mention, the kind whose names will mean nothing to the general population, and who have no opus to which other potential disciples can be directed. Often these are the people who have made the biggest difference to our lives.

One such hero in my life is a man called Dennis Cheeseman. He died recently, and he is particularly on my mind today, as I'm going to his memorial service tomorrow. Dennis was a schoolteacher and before that he flew in the RAF. But he was also a lobster and prawn fisherman, and this is the context in which I knew him, and remember him with great fondness.

Dennis lived in Osmington Mills, near Weymouth, and very near the holiday cottage which the parents of my best childhood friend, Charlie, rented for their summer holidays. Most years, from the age of about six to sixteen, I was invited to stay with the family, and we spent the best part of every day messing about on the beach at Ringstead Bay. Dennis kept his boat on the same beach. It was a beautiful wooden skiff, with a little outboard motor, perfect for his part-time, second occupation of working a few pots to catch crustacea to sell to local pubs and restaurants. And every time he came in from hauling his pots we'd crowd round to see what he'd caught.

Being a schoolteacher, Dennis was on holiday in the summer too. You'd have thought he'd had enough of kids, and that his potting was the perfect way to get away from them for a few weeks. But amazingly he responded to our goggle-eyed curiosity and prodding fingers by inviting us to come out with him on his boat, and help him pull his pots and sort his catch. To me the experience was sheer bliss. Every pot hauled was a lucky dip of wriggling and kicking marine fauna.

Spider crabs were something I'd never seen before, and looked suitably prehistoric to be credible sea monsters. But it was lobsters he was really after, and when he caught one we'd all cheer. Getting the tail-thrashing, claw-waving critters out of the pots with your bare hands was a dangerous mission for a seven-year-old. Dennis wouldn't let us try at first – no doubt he didn't relish the prospect of dropping us back on the beach with a digit or two less than we'd set out with. But by the time we'd been out with him a few times, and he'd shown us how to handle the creatures properly, we were trusted. It felt like promotion, and we began to think of ourselves less as passengers, and more as crew.

But the prawn pots were always my favourites. Dennis would

shake the contents out of them into a bucket, and when all the pots were hauled, he'd hand the bucket to us for sorting. We had to pick out the winkles, rockfish and tiny crabs. Our favourite thing to find was an astonishingly wriggly fish called a blenny. We were used to catching these in our nets in the rock pools on shore. But the ones in Dennis's pots were four or five times as big. We called them 'Cheesey size' in his honour, and they could give you a nasty nip – the kind that would make you scream but laugh at the same time. We'd put them in each other's boots or down our necks until Dennis would quietly tell us to pack it in, and make us chuck the poor thing overboard. He didn't mind fun and games, but he didn't like us being cruel for our own amusement.

And this was one of the great things about Dennis. He never made a big fuss about anything – but he didn't have to. He was the sort of person you naturally wanted to please, and he could always steer you in the right direction without ever raising his voice. Now that I have children of my own, I appreciate what a rare and delicate skill this is. It's the art of making those who look up to you feel good about themselves, and Dennis did it beautifully. It must have made him a great teacher.

I remember all this so well, because Charlie and I did this not once or twice, but many, many times. I don't quite recall how it came about, but what began as an occasional outing became a daily routine of the holiday. And not just for one summer, but year after year. For most of the children on the holiday, and there were often upwards of half a dozen in the cottage, going out with Dennis was an absolute high point. In the end a rota had to be drawn up to avoid fights about whose turn it was.

At least once every holiday, Dennis, his wife Pauline and daughter Caroline, would invite all of us from the cottage, adults and children, for a picnic on the beach outside his boat hut. He would cook us a batch of his prawns, boiling them in fresh water from a nearby stream. After draining them, he would put them back in the pan, add a handful of salt, and give them a shake. I've read many times since that the best way to cook live prawns is to boil them in heavily salted water or, better still, seawater. But Dennis's prawns were as sweet as anything. The salt got on to the prawns mainly from off your fingers, as you peeled them, and as a way of eating freshly gathered prawns it takes some beating.

I don't know much about the rest of Dennis's kitchen repertoire. But I do know that for my love of boats, of fishing, of the sea and its delicious harvest, and for the fact that I chose to make my life in West Dorset, I owe him a huge debt of gratitude.

When I made the first series of *River Cottage*, I asked Dennis if he would take me out to haul his prawn pots again, and if we could film it for the programme. Very sportingly, he agreed, and afterwards we had a prawn picnic by the boat hut one more time. It was only then, as I relived that childhood thrill in a more self-conscious, adult mode, that I realised that I learned as much from Dennis, about the importance of place, and people, in the pleasure of good food, as I ever did from Elizabeth David or Keith Floyd.

He is much missed, and will leave a Cheesey-size hole in the lives of all who knew him.

March 2005

Hugh's Quiz

This is based on the quiz I set for the *Guardian* in December 2004, although I have added a number of new questions for this collection to make it even more challenging!

The answers to this quiz can be found on the River Cottage website, rivercottage.net.

1) Medlars (the apple-like fruit of the medlar tree) are traditionally 'bletted' before being used in the kitchen. This means they are:

   a) soaked in beer

   b) covered in salt

   c) left to go a bit rotten

   d) passed through the digestive tract of a pig

2) In his *Complete Herbal*, Culpeper warns that peaches cause:

   a) lust

   b) piles

   c) hallucinations

   d) forgetfulness

3) Bannock-fluke is the old Scottish name for what?

   a) a haggis

   b) a smoked sausage

   c) a lucky biscuit

   d) a turbot

4) The common ingredient in dishes called Du Barry is:

a) prunes

b) leeks

c) cauliflower

d) truffles

5) Aristotle believed that elvers (baby eels) came spontaneously from where?

a) outer space

b) trees struck by lightning

c) the decomposing bodies of donkeys

d) the bowels of the earth

6) 'Chicken of the wood' is a colloquial name for a:

a) pheasant

b) yellow mushroom

c) large moth

d) cowardly gamekeeper

7) The deadly poison ricin can apparently be made at home from which of the following foods:

a) kidney beans

b) rice

c) cod liver oil

d) potatoes

8) Lord Archer's legendary Christmas parties always served:

a) bangers and mash and Bollinger

b) fish and chips and Veuve Clicquot

c) bubble and squeak and Dom Perignon

d) shepherd's pie and Krug

9) The most poisonous parts of the fugu (a puffer fish prized in Japan for the delicacy of its flesh as *sashimi*) are the:

a) fins

b) liver

c) reproductive organs

d) skin

10) During the war, 'mock grouse' was created by stuffing a kipper inside what?

a) a pigeon

b) a potato

c) a tin of corned beef

d) a pig's heart

11) What was the first canned fish?

a) the tuna in Florida in 1810

b) the sardine in Nantes in 1820

c) the pilchard in Cornwall in 1830

d) the salmon in Canada in 1840

12) Ethically speaking, you should not drink Campari if you are:

a) a vegetarian

b) a scientologist

c) on the pull

d) allergic to penicillin

13) According to the Goodies, the Lancastrian martial art of Ecky Thump involved striking your opponent with which food item?

a) a tin of spam

b) a giant leek

c) a wedge of cheese

d) a black pudding

14) The Greek wine retsina gets its distinctive taste from the addition of:

a) smoked fish roe

b) coal

c) pine resin

d) dead snakes

15) What was the affectionate food-related nickname of the legendary jazz-blues pianist whose real name was Ferdinand Lamothe?

a) Swiss Roll

b) Cheese Roll

c) Jelly Roll

d) Fig Roll

16) What kind of animal is a hogget?

a) a sheep

b) a pig

c) a fish

d) a bird

17) Falstaff, Peer Gynt and Oliver are all types of what?

a) Aigar

b) Brussels sprout

c) pickled herring

d) rolling pin

18) Who sang 'Life is a Minestrone'?

a) Tangerine Dream

b) 10cc

c) Daryl Hall and John Oates

d) The Soup Dragons

19) In 1840, a German philosopher and scientist by the name of Justus Liebig invented what?

   a) Oxo

   b) Bovril

   c) Marmite

   d) Bloater paste

20) The ugli fruit is the hybrid of a grapefruit and what?

   a) an orange

   b) a lemon

   c) a tangerine

   d) a lime

21) The officially recognised hottest chilli in the world was grown in:

   a) Texas

   b) Sri Lanka

   c) Dorset

   d) Mexico

22) What was Mrs Beeton's first name?

   a) Isabella

   b) Arabella

   c) Caramella

   d) Nigella

23) Ground elder is an edible weed, but it should not be consumed after it has begun to flower. Why?

   a) it becomes deadly poisonous

   b) it becomes hallucinogenic

   c) it becomes strongly laxative

   d) it makes you impotent

24) Soufflé Rothschild contains fruit macerated in a liqueur containing:

   a) gold

   b) frankincense

   c) myrrh

   d) cannabis

25) 'Age cannot wither her, nor custom stale her infinite variety: other women cloy the appetites they feed: but she makes hungry where most she satisfies.' Who was she?

   a) Helen of Troy

   b) Cleopatra

   c) Desdemona

   d) Fanny Craddock

26) Which Martin Scorsese film contains a lesson on the art of slicing garlic for a tomato sauce?

   a) *Mean Streets*

   b) *Casino*

   c) *Goodfellas*

   d) *The Last Temptation of Christ*

27) Which root veg did Uncle Monty in *Withnail and I* consider 'infinitely more beautiful than the rose'?

   a) the turnip

   b) the radish

   c) the carrot

   d) the swede

28) Yabba is the Australian for:

    a) toffee

    b) kangaroo meat

    c) mango

    d) crayfish

December 2004

INDEX

Advertising Standards Authority 29–30
Agas 255–7
agribusiness 131, 134–6
Al-Basha, Kensington 57
Alfredo's, Oxford 156
aphrodisiacs 56, 61, 63, 80
Armstrong, Elsiedale 235–6
Army ration packs 90–92
artisan food producers 232–3
Asda 146
asparagus 208–10
Atkins diet 21–4

baby food 213–14
Bacco, South Kensington 160–61
Bahamas 124–8
baked beans 202–3
Bando, Mitsugoro 78
Bareham, L., and Hopkinson, S. 267
bats 63, 66–7
Beck, Eric 46
beef on the bone 45–6, 211–13
Belben, Mike 167
Benamar, Kamel 169–70
Berry, Mary 255–7
Big Issue 144
biltong 60
biscuits 187–91, 220
Blair, Tony 132, 133
Bloody Mary 88–90
Blueprint Café, London 74
Blythman, Joanna 146–7
boar farming 233–7
Doden, Giles 89–90
Booth, Dr Derek 235
bouillabaisse 257–9
brains 44–6, 57, 71, 73–6, 237
Bramall, Lord 185

breakfast cereals 186–7
Bregoli, Mauro 240–41
British Academy of Gastronomes 183–5
British Wild Boar Association 235
Brown, Dr John 29, 30
Browning, Helen 109
BSE 44, 57, 71, 73, 75, 132, 137
Bull, Stephen 262–4
burger-plus restaurants 162–4
Bush, George 13, 137–8

Caine, Michael 180
Calvert, Harry 234–6
Calvin, Andrew 247
cannabis 93–4
Carluccio, Antonio 250
Carnivores, Nairobi 59
celebrity chefs 176–83
Celebrity Countdown (Channel 4) 95
cereal bars 31–3
chalet girls 42–3
Charlot, Roi des Coquillages 257–8
Château Petrus 96
Cheeseman, Dennis 268–71
chemicals 141–2, 145, 214
chickens, see poultry
child-friendly restaurants 199–201
children's cooking 195–7, 221–5
chitons 61–2
chocolate 217, 219–20
Christmas dinner 210–13
Clarke, Bob Carlos 178
Cleopatra Taverna, Notting Hill 171
Coats, Prue 67–9
Collingborne, Joe and Ro 109
Compassion in World Farming 106
concept restaurants 161–7
Connaught, London 45–6, 265–8

Cook on the Wild Side, A 55, 61
Country Weekenders 205–8
Creative Review 30
crème brûlée 242, 243–4, 267
crumbers 157–8
Cullen, Gary 118
Curtis, Tony 34

Daily Mail 141, 143, 177
David, Elizabeth 262–3, 268
Deals 162–3
Deighton, Len 184
Dieppe 253–5
diet industry 21–4, 25–7, 31–4
diving 83–4
Dobson, Frank 93
dogs 148–9
donkey salami 58
Dorchester, London 183–5
Dug Out 162
dunking 187–91

Eagle pub, Farringdon 167–8
eels 250–51
eggs 107, 237–9
Elsener, Willi 184
Erasmus, Udo 29
European Rail Catering 39
European Union 129–30
Eurostar 36–8
Evans, Gerard 90
Evening Standard 160
Eyre, David 167

factory farming 116, 117
    meat 70, 111, 113, 139
    poultry 19–20, 105–7
farm animals 114–16, 139–40
farm shops 145, 147, 153, 233, 236
fashion in food 153–6, 186
fast-food industry 3–20
fat 22, 25, 28–32
fat-free products 24–7, 31–2, 56
Fawlty Towers 228
fish 65–6
Fish! restaurant, London 165–7
fishing 112, 113, 118–31, 180, 198–9,
    206, 249
    fly 99–100, 129–31
    game 84–5, 118–23

Flora margarine 28–31
Floyd, Keith 268
food additives 143, 219
food-tasters 86–8
Forman, Marcel 246
Four Seasons, London 241
fox-hunting 110–12
France 231–2
Friends of the Earth 132
fruit 21, 22, 23, 247–9
fugu fish 62, 77–82

Gall, Sandy 184
game, African 59–60
gastro-pubs 167–8
George's, Oxford 204
giraffe 59
GM foods 131–8, 145
Golden Crackles 186
Good Food Guide 174, 176, 178,
    199
Goolden, Jilly 95
goose barnacles 62
gooseberries 248–9
Goosnargh corn-fed chicken 261
Gordon, Peter 243
government regulations 44–6, 57
Greek restaurants 171, 174–5
gulls' eggs 237–9

hangover cures 46–8
Harvey's, London 177, 179–80
Heathcote, Paul 260–61
Henderson, Fergus 70, 71
Hennequin, Denis 14
Henriques, Michael 245–7
Hero's, Oxford 204
High Cost of Low Price, The 18
Hirst, Damien 172, 173
Hole in the Wall, Bath 199
Holmbush Wild Boar Company 234–6
Hopkinson, S., and Bareham, L. 267
Hori, Ken-ichi 78–80
hydrogenated fats 28–9, 32

Iceland 129–31
impala 59
Independent on Sunday 93
insects 60–61
Istanbul Iskembecisi, London 44

Jaine, Tom 176–8
Joe's Brasserie, Wandsworth 88–90
Johnson, Allen 137–8
Johnson, Reg 260–61
junk food 15, 16, 19

Kellogg's 31–3, 186
Kentucky Fried Chicken 18–20
Kenya 118–23
kitchen tyrants 216–18
Koffman, Pierre 176–8
Korea 150

La Cantina 157
La Coupole, Paris 58
Lahore, Southall 75
Laperouse, Paris 95–7
Lapland 97–102
La Tante Claire, London 176–8
Lawson, Nigella 25–6, 144–5
Le Petit Blanc, Oxford 157
Les Alouettes, Claygate 177
Lichfield, Patrick 184
Linley, David 162
Little, Alastair 243, 244
local produce 144–6, 209, 260
Lola's, Islington 158
lone dining 159–61
L'Oranger, London 169–70
Loubet, Bruno 241–2
lunchboxes 218–21

Macaulay, Sean 8
McClancy, Jeremy 70
McDonald's 3–17, 55
MacLean, Norman 245–6
McVities 26–7
MAFF 44–5, 57, 71
maggots 60–61
margarine 28–31
Marmite Dieppoise 254
Maryland University 138, 140
Maschler, Fay 88, 202
Matthews, Bernard 19, 37, 56
Maynards 35
meat-eating 114–18
Monsanto 136
Moro, Exmouth Market 201
Morocco 39–41
Morris, Dave 14

Mosimann, Anton 184, 211
mushrooming 249–50

Nestlé: Golden Grahams 186–7
Newsnight (BBC TV) 137
Nontas, Camden 174–5
Novelli, Jean-Christophe 181–3

Oceanographic Institute 120
Odeon Cinemas 35
offal xi, 57, 70–71
OFM 154, 155
Old Manor House, Romsey 240–42
Oliver, Jamie 14
orchards 227–8
organic produce 134, 141–3, 214
Oxford University 202

Palosaari, Paivikki 98–102
pastilla 40–41
Paxman, Jeremy 138
Peat Inn, Fife 249
Permanent Global Summer Time 144–7
Perraud, Michel 177
Petri-meat 138–40
Pharmacy, Notting Hill 171–3
pigs 70, 111, 148–50
Pinneys of Scotland 246–7
plate-picking 48–51, 179
poultry 19–20, 105–7, 142, 260–61
Prewett Food: Dunkers 188–90
Private Eye 153–4, 25
processed foods 134, 142
Provence, Gordleton Mill 181
pub food 167–8
Punch 8, 88
Pusztai, Dr Arpad 137

railway food 36–9
Ramsay, Gordon 169
Randall Aubin, Soho 74
Ranga river, Iceland 130
Reading Scientific Services 86–8
recipes 71–3
    Fish soup 259
    Goosnargh corn-fed chicken 261–2
    Gulf gâteau 92
    Hash brownies 94
    Joe's Brasserie Bloody Mary 90
    Magaz (brain) curry 76

Mean beanz 203
Nettle soup 252–3
Quadruple chocolate chip cookies 27
Roast duck with lime compote 264–5
Slow-braised squirrel 69
reindeer 97–102
restaurants 156–85, 199–201, 240–42, 254, 265–8
retro menus 265–8
Ribena 33
River Cafe, Hammersmith ix–x, 57, 73, 241
River Cottage, Dorset 207–8
River Cottage (Channel 4) xii, 144, 271
River Cottage Cookbook, The 40
Riverside Restaurant, Dorset 200
Robinson, Adam 237
Ronay, Egon 184
rooks 58
Roux brothers 169
Rupert, Prince 59

St John Restaurant, London 71, 201
salmon 100, 130–31
Sanders, Colonel Harland 18–20
sandwiches 203–4
school meals 14, 17, 153, 218–21
Scotland 245–7, 249–50
sea urchins 62–3
seafood 61–3, 65–6,
Seafood Restaurant, Padstow 258
Seale, Mark 236–7
seasonality 144–8, 248
Seychelles 63, 65–7, 83–6
shooting 112, 113
Silcock, Bruce 60
slimming products 25–7, 32–3
smoked salmon 245–7
Sofianos, Aristodimos 185
Some Like It Hot 33
sprats 251–2
Spry, Constance 244
Spurlock, Morgan 14, 15
squirrel 58, 67–9, 117, 250
Star Inn, Harome 51
Steel, Helen 14
Stein, Richard 258

Sunday Times 257
Super Size Me 14, 15
supermarkets 17–18, 144, 145–7, 212, 232, 236
Superspread 29
sushi 85–6
Swaziland 59
Sweeney Todd's 162
sweeteners, artificial 33–4
sweets 35

tea-making 225–6
Tesco 17, 18
textured vegetable protein 140
Thames eels 250–51
Third World 134–6
Thomas, David 8
Tokyo 77–9
trans-fatty acids 28–31
transportation of food 144–5
Trebor 35
Trump, Ivana 179
Tudor Confectionery 35
tuna 42, 84–6
turkey 210–11

ume-sho bancha 47–8

Van den Bergh Foods 28–30
veal 107–10
vegans 108, 114
vegetables 24, 153–4, 214
vegetarians 114–16, 117, 140
Venner, James 239
Virgin Rail 39

Waddle, Chris 257
Wal-Mart 17, 18
warthog 59
water 158–9
Watson, Arthur 200
White, Marco Pierre 177, 178–80, 182
Whole Earth 29
Willet, Prof. Walter 28
Williams, David 234
wine 94, 204
Wodehouse, P. G. 46
woodlice 61
Wright, Simon 29

CREDITS

The publishers would like to thank the following publications for permission to reproduce the articles in this book:

Evening Standard: It's a McTaste crime, p.10; Dog's breakfast, p.31; The sour taste of sweet FA, p.33; Sweets gone sour, p.35; Telling porkies about bacon, p.38; Brainless, p.44; Spineless, p.45; Search for the golden crumber, p.157; Dear eau dear, p.158; Crème de la crème, p.243; Let's hear it for the green and hairy, p.247; Spring stingers, p.252. *Expressions*: Understanding Marco, p.178; Modest – moi?, p.181. *GQ Active*: Taste not, want not, p.55. *Guardian*: I'm lovin' it, p.13; Keeping it veal, p.107; The rhyme and reason of shopping in season, p.144; A silver miracle, p.251; Hugh's Quiz, p.273. *Independent*: Giving the Colonel his marching orders, p.18; Tunnelling new depths, p.36; Making a hash of it, p.93; No head for figures, p.94; When fish meets fashion, p.164; 'Waiter, are the acronyms fresh?', p.168; A good omen for Damien, p.171; Wild time in the New Forest, p.240; Grandeur in aspic, p.265. *Isis*: Service game, p.156; A hill of beans, p.202. *Observer*: Dr Death rides out, p.21; Fat free . . . and slightly lacking the brain department too . . . , p.24; A Moroccan pigeon's revenge, p.39; Confessions of a serial plate picker, p.48; If it swims or flies, eat it, p.65; Seychelles, sharks and sushi, p.83; A reindeer is not just for Christmas, p.97; Death of a chicken, p.105; Fox in a box, p.110; Vegetarians with teeth, p.114; Funeral for a fish, p.124; Scales of justice, p 129; Why GM will never feed the world, p.134; The petri-burgers are coming, p.138; Missing the point about organics, p.141; Of pigs and puppies, p.148; So what exactly is the new asparagus?, p.153; Playing with food, p.195; And that's just for starters, p.199; Ditch the bird for a happy Christmas, p.210; Baby food, p.213; Give me credit, p.216; Lunchbox jury, p.218; Pat a cake, pat a cake, p.221; My cup runneth over, p.225; The orchard of life, p.226; Locally produced to die for, p.231; Smoke signals from across the border, p.245; In memoriam: Dennis Cheeseman, p.268. *Punch*: Mac attack, p.3; Ski cuisine, p.41; Headcase, p.73; Panel eaters, p.86; Not bloody likely lads, p.88; The rations are coming, p.90; Oh solo me-o!, p.159; Bum deals, p.162; The Eagle has landed, p.167; It's all Greek to me, p.174; Snap, crackles and hype, p.186; First catch your dinner, p.249; Ferry fresh, p.253. *Sunday Express*: Murphy's law of genetic modification, p.131. *Sunday Telegraph*: Taking sides in the fat wars, p.28; Toasting Tufty, p.67; Heads or tails?, p.70; Use your brains, p.75; A fish to die for, p.77; Dunk food takes the biscuit, p.187; Taking the cure, instead of the car, p.205; Shelling out, p.237; Aga saga, p.255. *Sunday Times*: Does the hair of your dog bite?, p.46; Well done indeed!, p.176; Perfection – purely academic, p.183; Spears of joy, p.208; Wild in the woods, p.233; Fish soup opera, p.257; The cook of the north, p.260; The duck that made her ladyship grouse, p.262. *The Magazine*: Hooked by a tricky fish, p.198.

A NOTE ON THE TYPE

The text of this book is set in Bembo. This type
was first used in 1495 by the Venetian printer Aldus
Manutius for Cardinal Bembo's *De Aetna*, and was
cut for Manutius by Francesco Griffo. It was one of
the types used by Claude Garamond (1480–1561) as
a model for his Romain de L'Université, and so
it was the forerunner of what became standard
European type for the following two centuries.
Its modern form follows the original types
and was designed for Monotype in 1929.

Hugh's new book, *The River Cottage Fish Book* (written with Nick Fisher), will be published by Bloomsbury in October 2007.

www.bloomsbury.com